# Chicken Soup for the Soul
## Healthy Living:
### *Heart Disease*

Jack Canfield

Mark Victor Hansen

Vicki Rackner, M.D., F.A.C.S.
THE HOPE HEART INSTITUTE
UNIVERSITY OF WASHINGTON SCHOOL OF MEDICINE

**Health Communications, Inc.**
**Deerfield Beach, Florida**

*www.hcibooks.com*
*www.chickensoup.com*

We would like to acknowledge the many publishers and individuals who granted us permission to reprint the cited material.

*Drop Dead Gorgeous* reprinted by permission Tracey Conway. ©2004 Tracey Conway.

*The Angina Monologues* reprinted by permission Mark Christopher Drury. ©2003 Mark Christopher Drury.

*Life in the Fast-Food Lane* reprinted by permission Ruth Vance. ©2004 Ruth Vance.

*Ticked Off* reprinted by permission Rudy Wilson Galdonik. ©2004 Rudy Wilson Galdonik. Adapted from "Take Heart: True Stories of Life, Love and Laughter" ©2003 Rudy Wilson Galdonik.

*The Appointment* reprinted by permission Twink DeWitt. ©2004 Twink DeWitt.

*(Continued on page 132)*

**Library of Congress Cataloging-in-Publication Data**
**available from the Library of Congress**

©2005 Jack Canfield and Mark Victor Hansen
ISBN 0-7573-0271-8

Publisher: Health Communications, Inc.
3201 S.W. 15th Street
Deerfield Beach, FL 33442-8190

*Cover design by Larissa Hise Henoch*
*Inside book design by Lawna Patterson Oldfield*
*Inside book formatting by Dawn Von Strolley Grove*

# Contents

*Fear less, hope more,*
*eat less, chew more,*
*whine less, breathe more,*
*talk less, say more,*
*love more,*
*and all good things*
*will be yours.*

—Swedish Proverb

## Introduction:
## From the Heart

Your heart does its job, day in and day out, without a single, conscious thought from you. Take this moment to think about your heart.

What thoughts and images come to you? A heart-warming story. Your open-hearted, compassionate friend. How your first love won your heart and then left you brokenhearted. A heart-to-heart talk with your child. The time you had a change of heart. The charity that holds a special place in your heart. An artichoke heart. Advancing from "Go fish" to gin rummy to hearts. Your courageous leader who never lost heart. Playing a tune on the piano by heart. Learning to cut a heart from red construction paper. Your hand over your heart in salute to our country, or as a greeting or in gratitude.

Indeed, your heart is much more than a fist-sized organ that sits in your chest, a miraculous muscle that's divided into four chambers separated by four valves that work together under the direction of an electrical signal in a life-giving ballet that separates life from death.

This book offers stories about life, saving life,

mending broken hearts, sewing up holes in hearts, restarting quivering hearts and transplanting hearts in life's most generous gift of organ donation.

And this book offers lifesaving health information for anyone recovering from a heart attack, a stroke or any cardiovascular illness. We doctors are coming to understand that most of the factors that place you at risk for heart disease are under your control (although some are not). You shape your health with your moment-to-moment lifestyle choices.

We hope these stories warm your heart, and we hope that you take to heart your power in shaping your own health.

Vicki Rackner, M.D., F.A.C.S.
*The Hope Heart Institute*

♥

# Drop-Dead Gorgeous

*Nobody has ever measured,*
*even poets, how much the heart can hold.*

—ZELDA FITZGERALD

I've had my share of passionate stage kisses. As an actress, I've lip-locked with fellow thespians who have turned my knees to jelly and others who, frankly, could have used an extra strong Altoids®. Regardless of dreamy or seamy, I always knew my stage kisses were professional, not personal.

Until January 21, 1995. That night, it got deeply personal.

It wasn't a particularly romantic scene. We were at the close of a typical show. Our half-hour sketch comedy television series, *Almost Live!* had been on the air since 1984, and I was in my fifth year as a full-time writer-performer. Our national run on cable channel Comedy Central had vaulted us to new heights of popularity in our hometown of Seattle, and our audience that night was standing room only.

With the cast clustered tightly around our host, we waved good night *Saturday Night Live!*-style, and with applause ringing in our ears, the live taping ended. Waiting for an "all's clear" signal from our technical check, we took a couple of questions from the crowd.

Or at least that's what my colleagues told me we did. I have no memories of that show whatsoever. I do not recall anything that took place that day or for the several days that followed. Because that night, a minute or so after 10 P.M., I died.

Though I've written comedy for years, this is no joke. I have proof: the answer to Question 24 on my Seattle Fire Department Medical Incident Report, which asks "Patient Condition on Arrival." Two response options are provided: (1) Alive or (2) Dead. My report has a big circle around number two. I was dead. So it's official.

Witnesses say I stood onstage among my fellow actors, began to sway in a woozy-boozy fashion, murmured "I don't feel too . . ." then collapsed. The audience cracked up! Why wouldn't they? We had just performed a sketch spoofing the TV medical drama *ER*! They made the logical assumption it was simply an actor's pratfall, and a very skillful one, too. How could they know I was a victim of sudden cardiac arrest, resulting from a dangerously fast heart arrhythmia called ventricular fibrillation? No one dreamed a vibrant and healthy woman in her thirties would literally drop dead in front of them. But I did.

Fellow cast members knew my swoon wasn't part of the script. Rapidly it became clear this was not a simple faint. Our host, John, seeing my eyes roll up in my head, my ashen color and hearing the strangulated rasp known as agonal respiration (translation: dying breaths) escape my throat, turned to the crowd and shouted, "Does anyone have medical training?"

Amazingly, there were no health-care professionals in the audience. But far in the back, a young man built like a fireplug with close-cropped blond hair stood up and called out, "She looks like she might be having heart problems."

John beckoned to him, "Can you help her?" Without hesitation this young guy bounded down the aisle steps onto the set, knelt next to me, and thrust his index and middle fingers onto the side of my throat. Everyone froze in silence for several seconds.

Then he barked out, "Call 911!" and positioned my head, pinched my nose and sealed my parted lips with his mouth. Thus began our intense "make-out session," more commonly known as CPR.

My youthful leading man, Glen MacLellan, was a truck driver by day and a volunteer firefighter. He had never used his emergency CPR training until that night. Over and over he alternated between the "kiss" that sent oxygen-rich breath into my lungs and the rapid chest compressions that kept the blood moving and carried oxygen to my brain.

Following the initial flurry of fear and confusion, my colleagues and the audience propelled into action the Chain of Survival: The first question from the 911 dispatcher was, "Is someone administering CPR?"

"Yes!"

"Good—don't stop. We're sending a firefighter unit to you right away. Don't stop the CPR."

Though it seemed much longer to my friends, a fire truck was there in less than four minutes, followed by a paramedic EMS unit. They took over the CPR from Glen, intubated me to maximize respiratory efforts and prepped my chest for defibrillation. In layman's terms, they cut the clothes off my upper body, stuck a tube down my throat and applied paddles to the bare skin.

In the movies, the process of shocking a patient back to life is accomplished in about thirty seconds. In real life, it's a bit longer. I lay on the studio floor, clinically dead, for at least fifteen minutes. At 10:19 P.M., after more CPR, intravenous cardiac drugs and six— count 'em, six!—jolting shocks of increasing voltage from an automated external defibrillator (AED), paramedics restored a fragile, but viable heartbeat.

I joined the elite club of those who "come back." For an actress, it was the best "comeback" of my career. I am among the less than 5 percent of people worldwide who currently survive sudden cardiac arrest.

With the love and support of my family, friends and health-care professionals, I was released from the hospital eight days later, equipped with my own lifesaving equipment: an implantable cardioverter defibrillator (ICD) embedded firmly in my chest, monitoring every beat of my heart.

Now, about that "kiss." It was the most important in my life, onstage or off. And though Glen MacLellan was a complete stranger, and a young married father at that, I will never forget it or forget him. Even though I can't remember it at all.

Blanche DuBois's famous line that closes Tennessee Williams's poignant play *A Streetcar Named Desire* is "I have always depended on the kindness of strangers." Thanks to the kindness and bravery of a total stranger, I got a second chance at life.

When Glen and I met for the second time, it was once again on the set of *Almost Live!*, exactly two weeks after my sudden cardiac arrest. This time, it was me giving him a heartfelt hug and a tearful kiss. And there was no acting involved.

♥ *Tracey Conway*

# With Every Beat of Your Heart

Every day, your heart—a muscle about the size of your fist—beats over 100,000 times and pumps 2,000 gallons of blood to nourish the 60 trillion cells in your body.

The blood the heart needs to survive comes from two small arteries—the right and left coronary arteries. Each of these arteries has branches that supply blood to all areas of the heart. Electrical signals travel through the muscle fibers in your heart and cause contractions, which move blood in and out, in and out, second after second, minute after minute, day after day. Your amazing cardiovascular system orchestrates this rhythmic flow of blood throughout your body to bring life-giving oxygen to every single cell—and this delicate dance takes just about sixty seconds to complete its journey from the heart and back.

If blood doesn't get to a vital part of your heart, the muscle dies, the system suffers a loss of function and you may die. This type of blockage is the cause of death for more Americans, both men and women, than nearly all other causes combined—including cancer, accidents and diabetes.

Yet we don't often think about the technical details at all—unless, of course, you run up the stairs and feel your heart pumping in your chest or watch a scary movie and find your "heart in your throat." Or until something goes wrong.

Routine maintenance, however, can keep the system strong and healthy. Take your blood pressure. Get a cholesterol check and look at the fats flowing through your blood. And if you have a problem, don't ignore it out of fear or overconfidence. Lifestyle choices—what you eat, how much you exercise—can actually repair the residue from years of neglect and turn your system into a clean, sleek, pumping machine.

Every thirty-three seconds someone experiences a heart problem. Every minute someone dies. You don't have to be among these statistics.

Be heart smart. You can take control of your heart health. The good news is that prevention works—with every beat of your heart.

♥ *Think about* . . .
## am I at risk for heart disease?

Check your risk factors. (The rest of this book discusses how to reduce each of these risks for heart disease, a heart attack or a second heart attack.)

— Smoking

— High blood pressure

— High cholesterol

— Diabetes

— Overweight

— Inactivity

— Stress

— Family history of heart disease (you can't change your genes, but you can be vigilant)

The more risk factors you have, the more likely you are to have continuing heart disease and/or another heart attack. So don't ignore the problem—make lifestyle changes.

# My Page

My Thoughts _____

_____

_____

_____


My Feelings _____

_____

_____

_____


My Facts _____

_____

_____

_____


My Support _____

_____

_____

_____

♥

## The Angina Monologues

*In a full heart there is room for everything, and in
an empty heart there is room for nothing.*

—Antonio Porchia

We will all have that time in our lives when our knees buckle beneath us. That pink slip in your work mail slot. The phone call in the middle of the night. The "I don't love you anymore letter." The policeman at your door at 2 A.M. The heart disease diagnosis. How will you get through the next few hours, few days, few months, few years?

Here's how I did.

I was lap swimming at the YMCA and succumbed to chest pains and had to be rescued. I had pulled a muscle. Yeah, that's it.

At the hospital, they ruled out a heart attack. They were wrong. Three blood tests later, Doctor Doom came in the room to lower the boom. I had a myocardial infarction, a fancy name for what every man over forty fears most, a heart attack. After a cardiac dye test, Dr. Doom lowered the boom again. I needed a quadruple bypass. Now.

With an 8 A.M. surgery schedule, I spent a sleepless night alone crying. I had just lost ninety pounds but was still morbidly obese. I thought the surgery was a death sentence. My nurse, a young man named Thomas, convinced me to place myself in God's care. He told me to allow God, my family and friends to take care of me for ten days. On the eleventh day, he told me to take control again. It was great advice. I cried no more.

I recovered in record time. My rehabilitation was astounding. The doctor told me that losing those ninety pounds saved my life. If I had not lost that weight, he would have been unable to do the surgery. He would have given me medicine and sent me home to die. I have now lost a total of 170 pounds, and my life has zoomed into the stratosphere.

After heart surgery, I became fearless. Every day is now "gravy." I take nothing for granted anymore. I embrace family, friends, opportunities, challenges, fears and life. My friends call me "reMARKable."

Within three months, I had resumed my job, as well as swimming, strength training and my fitness transformation. I set new wild and seemingly insurmountable goals for a former 422-pound fat guy with a history of heart surgery. I went on radio and television to talk about reclaiming one's health. I became a certified aerobics instructor. I went 610 feet into the air parasailing over Disney World. I jumped from an airplane in a tethered skydive and parachuted 8,000 feet to the ground. I went from size 60 pants to wearing skimpy posing trunks onstage in a bodybuilding competition. YIKES!

I even discovered that I could sing. That's the remarkable thing about a lofty goal. Sometimes the fun is in the personal discoveries and growth along the way long before the goal ever comes into view.

I refuse to put limits on myself just because of my past. My past no longer dictates my future. I just won't allow it.

♥ *Mark Christopher Drury*

# Blood Pressure:
## Silent but Dangerous

Blood pressure goes up and down depending on your activities and emotions. But when it goes up and stays up all the time, you have a condition known as high blood pressure or hypertension.

The biggest problem with high blood pressure is that it usually has no symptoms. There is no way to know whether you have it unless you get your blood pressure measured and monitored regularly.

High blood pressure means your heart is working harder than normal—thus putting it and your coronary arteries under a greater strain. This eventually damages them. Uncontrolled high blood pressure can lead to:

- Hardening and thickening of the arteries
- Heart attack
- Stroke
- Congestive heart failure
- Impaired vision or blindness
- Kidney failure

A normal blood pressure is below 120/80. Anything over that could be a problem and should be watched or brought under control.

- Normal: below 120/80
- Pre-high blood pressure: 120/80 to 139/89 (You're at risk. Try diet and exercise to keep your numbers in the lower range.)
- High blood pressure: 140/90 or higher (In addition to lifestyle changes, you may need to take medication.)

The first number is your systolic, or pumping, pressure. The second number is your diastolic, or resting, pressure. Systolic is the beat of your heart, and diastolic is the pause between beats. The cuff wrapped around your arm allows the health-care provider to "hear" the rushing blood hitting the artery wall.

Lifestyle changes alone may get you back on track. These include weight loss with a low-fat diet with at least eight to ten daily servings of fruits and vegetables and about three servings per day of low-fat dairy; cutting back on salt; regular, brisk exercise; stress management; and restricting or avoiding alcohol. If these don't lower your blood pressure, medication can help.

## How to Take Your Blood Pressure at Home

Blood pressure recorded in the doctor's office is often not an indicator of your blood pressure's actual response to the "real world."

Nervousness about having your blood pressure taken can cause it to rise—a condition known as "white coat" hypertension. So monitoring your blood pressure at home may give you and your doctor a more accurate picture of your actual reading.

Always have more than one measurement of your blood pressure in different places, especially if your doctor recommends you take medication. And take your home monitor to your doctor's office and make sure it gets the same reading as your doctor's monitor.

For a more accurate reading:

- Avoid caffeine, cigarettes and alcohol for thirty minutes before you take a reading.
- Relax for three to five minutes.
- Sit down with your legs and ankles uncrossed and back supported.
- Make sure to use correct cuff size. Large people need a larger cuff.
- Place your arm on a table so that your arm cuff is at the level of your heart and your arm is at a 90-degree angle to your body. The bottom edge of the cuff should be one inch above the crease of your elbow.
- Keep a record of your blood pressure readings, noting the time of day.

## ♥ Think about . . .
### questions to ask my doctor

♥ What is my blood pressure reading in numbers? (Write this down and keep track of your readings.)

♥ What is my goal blood pressure?

♥ Is there a healthy eating plan I should follow to help lower my blood pressure and lose weight? (A suggested DASH diet is described in this book.)

♥ Is it safe for me to do regular physical activity? (Most of the time, your doctor will encourage you to do regular activity.)

♥ What is the name of my blood pressure medication? What is the generic name?

♥ What time of day should I take my blood pressure medicine?

♥ Should I take it with or without food?

♥ What should I do if I forget to take my blood pressure medication at the recommended time?

♥

# Life in the Fast-Food Lane

*Anybody who believes that the way to a man's
heart is through his stomach flunked geography.*
—ROBERT BYRNE

Don't get me wrong. My husband isn't obese. But he's just topped fifty years old, and he's carrying what seems to be the obligatory (for middle-aged men) fifteen or twenty extra pounds around the waist. He says it's his "survival pack" in case he gets lost in the desert, but we don't live anywhere near a desert, and I know they have a snack bar on the golf course.

Meanwhile, his cholesterol isn't dangerous (yet), but it's on the high end of safe. His blood pressure isn't what it used to be. And all those triglycerides I keep hearing about . . .

His doctor says he needs to get his numbers down, which wakes me up in the middle of the night with cold sweats but seems to have, somehow, had little to no effect on the person who could actually be harmed.

Plus the man has some bad habits. One night he went to the grocery store and came back with a box of chicken legs that was on such a "great sale" he just had to buy it, which of course means it was so old they legally had to throw it out in another fifteen minutes. That's why they were practically giving it away. He sat down in front of the television and ate the whole box—even though we had only eaten dinner half an hour before.

All of which means I was pleasantly surprised when he seemed to take to my new diet. It wasn't a radical diet; I just started cooking a little more health-consciously. I served smaller portions of meat and filled out the plate with more vegetables. I tried new recipes that focused on healthier choices instead of pork chops and gravy (his favorite). I stopped buying soda and chips because I knew if they were anywhere in the house my husband would find them. One time, I even replaced the ground beef in my homemade tacos with beans. Maybe that was pushing it, but I only did that once.

For a while, he complained. He was hungry all the time. The portions were too small (because the vegetables apparently didn't count). There wasn't anything in the pantry for his after-dinner snack. I didn't argue, but I didn't change my approach either. This wasn't just a whim; this was for our health. I didn't want to be a widow in my fifties or sixties like two of my friends.

Eventually he came around. He never tried to eat

his vegetables, but he stopped complaining. He stopped rummaging through the pantry after dinner. He even stopped buying that day-old chicken.

I was feeling pretty good about our new lifestyle until the day I was driving his car and had to slam on the brakes to avoid an accident. Out from under the seat rolled an empty Mountain Dew can. I pulled over and took a closer look.

The space underneath the seat was crammed with soda cans and Whopper wrappers. My learning-to-eat-healthy-so-he-wouldn't-have-a-heart-attack husband had been regularly indulging in an "appetizer" before dinner.

I haven't entirely stopped trying to live healthy (still no chips in the house), but I've gone back to steak and pork chops for dinner (smaller portions, trimmed the fat). It seems like a fair compromise . . . for now.

♥ *Ruth Vance*

# Cholesterol: It's All in the Numbers

Blood cholesterol is a soft, waxy, fatlike substance found in your blood and in all cells of your body. Unhealthy blood cholesterol levels are one of the major risk factors for heart disease—and a key measure your doctor will monitor to prevent you from having a heart attack.

Healthy adults should have their blood cholesterol and triglyceride levels measured at least once every five years. If you are recovering from a heart attack, your levels should be measured much more often.

## Eleven Great Ways to Get Your Blood Cholesterol Under Control

1. **Exercise.** Walk, run, bike, swim or otherwise get yourself moving for at least thirty minutes most days of the week. Exercise can help raise "good" HDL levels.
2. **Lose excess weight.**
3. **Drink alcohol in moderation** if at all. One or two drinks a day may help raise "good" HDL levels, but alcohol is high in calories and increases the risk of high blood pressure.
4. **Don't smoke.**
5. **Eat less saturated fat.** This is the type found in animal foods. Saturated fat has a far more

negative impact on your blood cholesterol than the dietary cholesterol found in foods such as eggs.

6. **Limit foods made with partially hydrogenated** (hardened) **vegetable oils.** These foods contain artery-clogging saturated and trans fats. Examples are store-bought cookies and crackers, vegetable shortening (use olive oil) and margarines.

7. **Choose artery-friendly monounsaturated fats** (such as olive oil and canola oil).

8. **Eat fish** once or twice a week for its heart-healthy omega-3 fats. Green leafy vegetables such as spinach and broccoli, as well as walnuts and flaxseed, also contain omega-3s.

9. **Eat more fiber** in fruits, vegetables and whole grains. Make sure the bread label says 100 percent whole wheat flour as the first ingredient. Eat less sugar.

10. **Be happy and make time to relax.** Anger and hostility have been linked to heart disease. Get enough sleep. Take regular breaks from your routine. These are called vacations. Learn a relaxation technique such as meditation.

11. **Talk to your doctor.** Discuss how you can make diet and other lifestyle changes to see how they affect your blood chemistry. Cholesterol-lowering medication is available, but try lifestyle changes first.

♥ *Think about . . .*
my cholesterol

## TOTAL BLOOD CHOLESTEROL LEVEL

The lower the better      My level ____

| Below 200 | Desirable |
| 200 to 239 | Borderline high |
| 240 or greater | High |

## HDL CHOLESTEROL LEVEL

The higher the better      My level ____

| 40 or greater | Desirable |
| Under 40 | Not desirable |

## LDL CHOLESTEROL LEVEL

The lower the better      My level ____

| Under 70 | Desirable for those at very high risk* |
| Under 100 | Desirable for those at high risk* |
| Under 130 | Desirable |
| 130 to 159 | Borderline high |
| 160 or greater | High |

*For anyone at moderate to high risk for heart disease, especially those who have had a heart attack, chest pain, angioplasty, bypass surgery, obstructed blood vessels, diabetes, among other risk factors

## TRIGLYCERIDE LEVEL

The lower the better      My level ____

| | |
|---|---|
| Under 150 | Normal |
| 150–199 | Borderline high |
| 200–499 | High |
| 500 or higher | Very high |

### Grocery Shopping

Want to control your cholesterol?
Read food labels and buy foods low in
saturated fat and low in cholesterol.
Here's a shopping list:

- ♥ Whole wheat, rye or pumpernickel
  bread
- ♥ Soft tortillas (corn or whole wheat)
- ♥ Hot and cold cereals, except gra-
  nola or muesli
- ♥ Grains (bulgur, couscous, quinoa,
  barley, hominy, millet rice)
- ♥ Fruits (any fresh, canned, dried or
  frozen without added sugar)
- ♥ Vegetables (any fresh, frozen or
  low-salt canned without cream
  or cheese sauce)

- ♥ Fresh or frozen juices, without added sugar
- ♥ Fat-free or 1 percent milk
- ♥ Cheese (with 3 grams of fat or less per serving)
- ♥ Low-fat or nonfat yogurt
- ♥ Lean cuts of meat (eye of round beef, top round, sirloin, pork tenderloin)
- ♥ Lean or extra lean ground beef
- ♥ Chicken or turkey (remove skin)
- ♥ White meat fish
- ♥ Tuna (light meat canned in water)
- ♥ Peanut butter (reduced fat)
- ♥ Eggs, egg whites, egg substitutes
- ♥ Low-fat cookies or angel food cake
- ♥ Low-fat frozen yogurt, sorbet, sherbet
- ♥ Popcorn, pretzels, baked tortilla chips
- ♥ Vegetable oil (canola, olive, corn, peanut, sunflower)
- ♥ Nonstick cooking spray
- ♥ Sparkling water, tea, lemonade

♥

## Ticked Off

*What comes from the heart, goes to the heart.*

—SAMUEL TAYLOR COLERIDGE

The FBI was about to be called in; the parking garage was already surrounded. Then suddenly I turned and saw it—a tidal wave bearing down on me. Drowning me. I gulped for air. I was doomed.

I woke with a start, happy to find it was all a dream. But as the vision of a tidal wave washed away into the recesses of my mind, the sensation of drowning did not. Sitting up, gasping for breath, I wondered why in the world I was still feeling the effects of a dream. There was gurgling in my chest. As I inhaled harder and deeper to bring fresh air to my lungs, it was clear that this wasn't just some awful dream. It was time to report a woman overboard.

One of the downsides of being a chronic emotional lunatic is the crying-wolf syndrome. The more lunacy you weave into your days, the less likely people who live with you will be willing to jump up in the middle of the night to throw you a life preserver. A gentle nudge and a whisper in my husband's ear only garnered a grumble and a wave of the hand. I needed to call in the generals.

"Dr. Shurman, an amazing thing happened last night," I told my cardiologist on the phone the next morning. "I drowned in bed."

"How soon can you get in?"

"In? You want me to make an appointment?" I just wanted to chat. I wanted to be told, "Hey, no problem. Drowning is not a biggie. Take two aspirin, and you'll be as good as new in a jiffy." I didn't like the drop-everything-and-get-your-butt-in-here attitude.

Only moments after a quick listen with the stethoscope, Dr. Shurman announced that I was in cardiac failure. Oh, please. Not that I wanted to butt in and tell Dr. Shurman his business, but if there's one thing I know it's words, and the word *failure* in the dictionary means a state of inability to perform.

The mere fact that I was sitting in his office chatting away would suggest that my heart was doing exactly what it was supposed to.

But Dr. Shurman was stubborn. He was not going to be swayed, and he even went so far as to suggest his understanding of my insides was a bit more on the money than mine. To prove his point, he ordered an echo test.

An echo test is one of my personal favorites. Lie still on a gurney while some tech smears jelly all over you and then produces amazing pictures on a computer screen, all with a wave of a microphone wand. Yes, an echo would be fine.

Soon after the echo, a powwow was called—perhaps, as Dr. Shurman suggested, to provide the most well-rounded medical expertise for my quirky and very sick heart.

Open-heart surgery, they pronounced. It seemed endocarditis bacteria bugs had been chewing on my heart months earlier, and this, combined with years and years of wear and tear, meant I needed not one but two of my valves replaced.

I was scheduled for a cardiac catheterization. A test that appears grizzly on paper is, with the right mix of happy drugs, not even a close second to the torment that can reign in a dentist's chair.

Shortly thereafter, my heart surgeon explained what lay in store. He held out a paperweight in which a mechanical heart valve was embedded. It looked like two metal doors swinging off hinges, attached to a fuzzy white ring. This piece of apparatus, which would extend my life, looked more like it belonged inside a toilet rather than in the human heart. But who was I to argue? As a repeat open-hearter (I was born with a hole in my heart), I didn't have any trouble getting to the heart of the matter.

"Drugs, I want drugs."

"Don't worry, we're fully capable of managing pain."

"No, I want way more than managed pain. I want to be happy. And no respirator. I don't like respirators."

"Well, you will wake up on a respirator, but we'll take it out as soon as you are able to breathe on your own." I made a mental note: fight the respirator (a really stupid plan I learned later).

After the surgery, too weak to move, too groggy to care, I just hung out in intensive care recovery, desperately trying to grasp bits of conversation.

"What do you think you're doing?" No longer impaled on a respirator, but suffering the effects of my futile attempts to spit it out, I was only able to rasp to a resident who was heading in my direction.

"Huh?" the startled resident asked. "I'm going to take a listen."

"Oh, no, you're not. I just watched you sneeze into your hand and then wipe it on a towel. You think you're coming anywhere near me?" With eyes bulging, this anonymous resident turned to the sink and slowly scrubbed his hands, over and over.

My homecoming was quiet except for the very reason I was in the hospital in the first place. My new heart valves, which were metal doors (or rather, highly polished pyrolytic carbon leaflets), banged shut every time they were called to service, which was with every beat of my heart. This produced a sound just like the ticking of a time bomb.

If everything was quiet, anyone could hear me ticking.

Frankly, I found the whole thing creepy, which I promptly reported to my heart surgeon. He told me, "It'd be really creepy if you didn't hear ticking, because you'd be dead." Which I guessed was some sort of consolation.

Eventually the ticking provided a unique opportunity. I found that the sound was amplified in certain places, most notably public restrooms. Once as two women did their thing in a highway rest stop bathroom, one of the women picked up on the strange sound.

"You hear that?" the lady asked her friend.

"Yeah, whaddya think it is?"

"Gee, sounds like a clock," I interjected. They must have agreed because both women held their digital watches up to their ears. But if it wasn't a clock, what could it be?

By the time I had completed my bathroom procedure, the two women were mapping out an all-encompassing hunt into every corner of the restroom. I just hoped they weren't planning on calling in bomb-sniffing dogs.

♥ *Rudy Wilson Galdonik*

# The Diabetes Connection

Diabetes more than doubles the risk of heart disease. Adding other risk factors to diabetes (such as smoking, unhealthy blood cholesterol levels, high blood pressure) has an enormous negative impact on your cardiovascular system.

About a third of the 16 million Americans who have diabetes don't know it. They are not only at risk for heart attack and stroke, but they risk other serious complications.

Type 2 diabetes tends to appear in middle age and among people who are overweight and inactive. In its mild form, diabetes can go undetected for many years. But uncontrolled diabetes greatly increases your risk of heart disease.

The keys to controlling diabetes or preventing it from developing are many of the same strategies for living a heart-healthy lifestyle:

- Maintain a healthy weight.
- Make healthy food choices.
- Keep your blood sugar level (glucose level) under control and monitor yourself regularly with your doctor.
- Watch for symptoms that might signal diabetes such as excessive thirst, extreme hunger or fatigue, unexplained weight loss, blurry vision,

frequent urination, skin infections, slow healing of cuts and drowsiness.

## Tests for Diabetes

Your doctor can perform two simple
blood tests to check for diabetes:

- ♥ A **blood glucose** (also called blood
  sugar) reading taken with a glucose
  monitor using a drop of blood can
  instantly check your blood sugar
  level at one point in time. High
  levels indicate diabetes or risk for
  diabetes and the need for further
  testing.
- ♥ A more complex blood test called
  the **hemoglobin A1C** measures
  your average blood glucose levels
  over the last three months. A high
  level may confirm the diagnosis of
  diabetes.

♥

## The Appointment

*A cheerful heart is good medicine.*
—Proverbs 15:13

In the sterile exam room, my husband, Denny, and I waited for the cardiologist. Because of Denny's weakness and exhaustion, a technician had readjusted his pacemaker just before Christmas in 1997. As the new year began, the doctor would give us the results of his follow-up tests and explain my husband's constant fatigue.

When the cardiologist entered, he shuffled papers, sat on the edge of his chair and looked at my fifty-year-old husband. "You've developed hypertension. You're still in atrial fibrillation." He hung his head and continued, "And you have hypertrophic cardiomyopathy." I couldn't reach Denny's hand, but our eyes locked. The doctor's body language frightened me.

"What's car . . . dium pathy?" I stumbled over the word.

Our doctor showed us the tiny echocardiogram images.

"What's the prognosis?" I asked. He shrugged his shoulders. He put Denny on antihypertensive medication and sent us home.

That afternoon we searched the Internet to learn more about cardiomyopathy—a severe weakening of the heart tissue. We found that this serious disease enlarges the heart, stretches and weakens it, often causing irregular heartbeats and other serious problems. In 1998 all treatment decisions seemed to end in heart transplant.

What did this mean for our lives? Denny, a missionary dentist, served with Mercy Ships and planned to lead a dental team to El Salvador in February. Could we continue in this work we both loved? After extended prayer, we believed we should go to El Salvador. The doctor approved.

Within weeks we unloaded equipment from the ship and set up the dental clinic. A few days later streams of grateful patients came to the clinic where they received restorations, extractions and loving concern from the team. I noticed Denny's fatigue, but the joy of working and praying with patients spurred him on.

While we were there, the Mercy Ships medical department conducted a one-week physicians' seminar on board. Doctors from El Salvador heard specialists from the United States present practical, up-to-date information.

As we ate lunch, the physicians came into the ship's dining room. Denny told me, "I hear there's a cardiologist here for the seminar. Sure would be good to talk to him."

Two minutes later a handsome young man asked, "Mind if I join you?"

"Please do," Denny extended his hand as he read the nametag, *Dr. Jeff Carr, Cardiologist.* He swallowed hard and proceeded with a casual conversation. "Where are you from?"

"Tyler, Texas." He smiled.

Denny put both arms on the table, shook his head as if to make sure he had heard correctly and said, "So are we."

The discussion that followed revealed Dr. Jeff's favorite seminar topic: cardiomyopathy. Denny had questions, and the cardiologist answered them all. As the two stood to go back to work, they shook hands. "Call my office as soon as you get back to Texas," Dr. Jeff said.

Three weeks later my exhausted husband and I walked into the friendly office of Dr. Jeff Carr. After a thorough workup and extensive tests, he changed Denny's medication and outlined foods to avoid.

Denny's health improved, and soon it was time for a cardioversion—a procedure in which the physician uses paddles to administer direct current to stop the atrial fib (just like on *ER*). When the heart began a normal rhythm after the first attempt, I saw Dr. Jeff shake his head and grin.

A few months later an angiogram startled the medical team. Dr. Jeff explained, "The ventriculargram aspect shows his heart has actually grown stronger."

We couldn't believe it. My husband went from a devastating diagnosis to a healthier life. How did it happen? Prayer, a divine appointment and the expertise of a compassionate physician combined to prove that a heart transplant is not the only answer to cardiomyopathy.

♥ *Twink DeWitt*

# Two Opinions Can Be
# Better Than One

Are you having chest pain or symptoms of heart disease, but your doctor can't nail down a diagnosis? Are you newly diagnosed with a heart condition? Are you among the lucky two-thirds who have survived a first heart attack? Are you confused about what the doctors are telling you about your heart? Do you fully understand the medical decisions you are being asked to make? Does the treatment plan make sense to you?

Consider getting a second opinion from another doctor if . . .

- Your doctor is unable to make a definite diagnosis within three visits, and symptoms don't go away.
- Your doctor says you have a serious, chronic or potentially fatal heart condition.
- Your doctor recommends surgery.

## ♥ *Think about . . .*
## questions to ask about my diagnosis

Ask these questions. Take notes. Share your thoughts, fears and feelings.

- ♥ What is wrong? What is my diagnosis?

- ♥ How serious is this?

- ♥ What caused this problem? (Is it something I did or did not do?)

- ♥ Can I prevent this problem from happening again? How?

- ♥ Are tests needed? Which ones?

- ♥ How will the results of these tests be helpful to me?

- ♥ Are there risks associated with these tests? What risks?

- ♥ Is treatment needed? What treatment?

- ♥ How effective is this treatment for conditions such as mine?

- ♥ Are there any treatment alternatives?

- ♥ Are there any treatment side effects?

- ♥ How will this treatment affect me physically, mentally and emotionally?

- ♥ How long will I have to have this treatment?

- ♥ Will there be any pain?

- ♥ What is your plan if the treatment does not work?

- ♥ Should I see a specialist such as a cardiologist or neurologist?

- ♥ Should I get a second opinion?

## My Page

My Thoughts _____

_____

_____

_____

My Feelings _____

_____

_____

_____

My Facts _____

_____

_____

_____

My Support _____

_____

_____

_____

♥

## Kicked Off the Merry-Go-Round

*It's not stress that kills us; it is our reaction to it.*
—HANS SELYE

It sneaked up on me ever so slowly, like a wave, and then, all of a sudden, it washed over me. Oh, I'd noticed that my clothes were fitting a little snugger, but, of course, I thought they'd probably shrunk a little during laundering (we fool ourselves in so many ways when we don't want to face the truth). And I noticed that I was a little out of breath when I walked up the stairs or went for a walk, but it was only "just a little."

And about that heartburn—last time I had it was when I was pregnant (and I knew I wasn't pregnant!). "Boy, it's hell to get old," I told my peers, as we jokingly compared our latest aches and pains.

I was trying to keep up with the hectic pace of life (yet I was slowing down), running a business, spending time with family, volunteering and keeping up with responsibilities at home. So much to do, so little time. I felt like I was on a merry-go-round!

A disagreement with a client was the incident

that took me beyond my ability to cope. Not long
after this conflict, I began experiencing neck pain
that resembled a charley horse. Then I began having
difficulty breathing and severe pain in my head. I
privately denied that these warning signs were anything serious and attributed the discomforts to the
stress in my life. I said to myself, *Relax, don't worry,
these pains will go away.* But within the next two
weeks, the episodes of discomfort escalated.

During one of the episodes of neck pain and
breathing difficulty, my husband took a hard look
at my face and took matters into his own hands.
"I'm taking you to the ER," he said. I made no
protest, secretly relieved that he had made the decision for me.

True to the way things usually work, the pain
had subsided by the time we got to the hospital. In
spite of that, I submitted to an EKG, blood tests
and long periods of waiting. The doctor finally
returned with the results of the tests and said with
raised eyebrows, "This is a bit of a surprise." Indeed
it was. She admitted me for more tests because my
heart enzymes were slightly elevated. Elevated
heart enzymes? I had heard of this . . . and it scared
me to death.

From that point on, everything became a hazy,
gray blur. I don't recall much of what transpired
during the next few days. I was told that the doctors

planned to perform an angiogram as well as an angioplasty. But the next morning, twenty minutes into the procedure, the surgeons realized that my condition was worse than they'd expected—a triple bypass was necessary. But it was Memorial Day, and a complete surgical staff was not available, so I was kept sedated until the *following* morning when the whole operating team would be on deck.

I don't recall what transpired during those lost days, but through conversations with family, some of the blank spots have been filled. I spent seven more days in the hospital before I could go home to start my healing process.

Without my family and friends sitting vigil in my room, the recovery would have been even more difficult. During my nine days in the hospital, a blur of people streamed in and out of my room day and night. Someone weighed me every morning, tested my blood every hour and brought my meds. And I saw a variety of doctors: three different primary-care physicians, two cardiologists, my surgeon, a dietitian, a wound specialist, my endocrinologist and a cast of others, not counting a host of nurses who changed every shift.

My nurse Tyler took care of me three long shifts in a row, so we had a chance to get acquainted. He made a huge difference in my recovery at "Spa St. Vincent's" (our nickname for the hospital).

One day, he brought fresh towels and clean "jammies," announcing that it was time to take a shower. I think I was starting to smell. As he helped me to the bathroom, I looked up at him coyly and said, "I used to be pretty hot stuff!" We shared a good laugh, because I certainly didn't look like "hot stuff" at that particular moment with no makeup, my hair flattened to my head and my tush hanging out the back of the skimpy hospital gown. We found something to laugh at every day. Tyler was one of the many angels in my steady journey toward health.

With this second chance to live, I continue to reevaluate my priorities. I've always coexisted with joy and a positive attitude, but I wasn't taking care of my health. Now, it's imperative that I make sensible life choices because if I don't have my health, I have nothing. Like many people, I needed a "wake-up call." Don't wait until something awful happens. *Learn from my experience and take charge of your own life.*

♥ *Jan Richardson*

## Lessen the Stress

If someone cuts you off in traffic, do you yell? Give them hand signals?

If you're in the ten-items-or-fewer checkout lane at the grocery store, do you get angry if the person in front of you has thirteen items?

If so, you have a hot button, and that is not good from a heart-health standpoint. The way we respond to life's stresses may predict who might have a heart attack. People who are highly depressed, angry, hostile, socially isolated, have lost a spouse or live alone are at a much higher risk for heart attack.

Are you a hot reactor? Quick-tempered? Or is your anger on slow simmer? An incident that makes your "blood boil" or causes you to "fly off the handle" can spike your blood pressure. Add to that a rush of stress hormones such as cortisol, and you could turn yourself into a walking time bomb that triggers chest pain leading to a heart attack.

If you turn to alcohol, cigarettes and fatty foods for stress relief, you will increase your heart disease risk. That is certain.

A far better bet is to use regular brisk exercise and relaxation techniques such as meditation to reduce tension, frustration, anxiety and worry.

## The Up Side of Stress

Not all stress is bad. The body has an amazing ability and some powerful brain chemicals called endorphins to put you back in control.

The challenges of life are often pleasant, and as the father of stress, Hans Selye, says, "Stress is the spice of life." Some things are just plain good, such as successfully completing a task, a thrilling ride in an amusement park or friendly competition.

When you have that "winning" feeling, you are experiencing the good parts of stress. Cardiologist Dr. Robert Eliot liked to tell the story about a coroner who told him, "I've never been called to a racetrack and asked to examine a body that was clutching a winning ticket."

Winners spark the release of brain chemicals that make you feel good—more powerful than morphine. It's our built-in reward system. Attempt tasks that make you feel like a winner. Your heart will be happier.

## ♥ Think about . . .
## how well I deal with stress

Indicate how strongly you agree with each of the following statements:

4 = all of the time;  3 = often;  2 = sometimes; 1 = never

\_\_\_\_ I am regularly exhausted by daily demands at work and home.

\_\_\_\_ My stress is caused by outside forces beyond my control.

\_\_\_\_ I am trapped by circumstances that I just have to live with.

\_\_\_\_ No matter how hard I work to stay on top of my schedule, I never feel caught up.

\_\_\_\_ I have financial obligations I cannot meet.

\_\_\_\_ I dislike my work but cannot take the risk of a career change.

\_\_\_\_ I'm dissatisfied with my personal relationships.

\_\_\_\_ I feel responsible for the happiness of people around me.

\_\_\_\_ I am embarrassed to ask for help.

_____ I do not know what I want out of life.

_____ I am disappointed that I have not achieved what I had hoped for.

_____ No matter how much external success I have, I feel empty inside.

_____ If the people around me were more competent, I would be happier.

_____ Many people have let me down in the past.

_____ I "stew" in my anger rather than express it.

_____ I am enraged and resentful when I am hurt.

_____ I can't take criticism.

_____ I am afraid I'll lose my job.

_____ I do not see the value of expressing sadness or grief.

_____ I do not trust that things will work out.

_____ TOTAL NUMBER OF POINTS

SCORING:

| | |
|---|---|
| 80-70 | Life has become one crisis and struggle after another. |
| 69-50 | Your options are often clouded, and you feel trapped. |
| 49-30 | You have an awareness that your life is in your hands. |
| 29-20 | You are your own best ally with a high degree of control, self-esteem and identity. |

♥

## Singing His Heart Out

*Wheresoever you go, go with all your heart.*

—CONFUCIUS

"All right, folks," my father-in-law announced, "our last song for today is *I Can't Stop Loving You.*" After my keyboard introduction, he opened up with the melting tones of his tenor sax. Then my husband, Don, began singing in his glorious baritone.

This was a big day for eighty-seven-year-old Oliver Hanson, who just the winter before had wed his seventy-seven-year-old bride after both lost their former mates. Now for Father's Day, dozens of relatives from both sides converged on the newly-weds for a let's-get-acquainted celebration. Since my father-in-law still played three musical "gigs" a week, he decided this joyous occasion called for a concert by one of his groups, "Donnie, Bon and Dad"—that is, my husband, myself and Oliver.

For most of Don's life, he and his father had been estranged. Only in the last few years had his father reached out to him. So today my fifty-nine-year-old husband was singing his heart out in gratitude. Plus hitting the highest notes possible on his trumpet, despite playing outdoors in 100-degree-plus heat.

After that song, everyone headed indoors for a potluck buffet. Everyone, that is, except for Don. Where was he?

Alarmed, I rushed from room to room. Suddenly he staggered out of one of the bathrooms—*in the midst of a massive heart attack.* He had literally "sung his heart out"—his last high notes triggering a clot that hit scar tissue in one of his arteries. A scar left over from childhood scarlet fever.

According to the emergency room physician, their only hope was to give Don streptokinase. "With it," he explained, "there's a 10 percent chance he'll survive. Without it, zero."

Terrified at the thought of losing Don, I replied, "Doctor, let's try it and pray that it works." My husband did survive. But half his heart was destroyed forever.

Told by his doctor that medication and exercise were his only hope, Don began a rigorous regime of biking—up to three hours daily. Even so, he soon ended up in the emergency room with a v-tach (ventricular tachycardia). As the months went on, such "events" came weekly, often daily.

Then one November day he was biking as usual near our home, when—blackout. *Sudden cardiac death!*

The next thing he remembers was being on the grass near the curb with a crashed bike, shattered glasses, badly dented helmet—and paramedics all around. It just so happened that our town's Christmas Parade was scheduled that day on an adjacent street, a parade including these same paramedics.

When a passerby saw Don fall, she dialed 911, and they rushed to his aid.

The good news is that the paramedics' special shocking equipment jolted his heart back into action. The bad news was having his heart stop in the first place, causing that crash.

Obviously, medicine and exercise alone weren't enough. Desperate, Don decided to be proactive. On his own, he began intense research in medical books and sought more doctors' opinions. That's how he discovered artificial implantable defibrillator devices (now called "generators"), created to help critical heart patients such as himself.

After verifying their effectiveness with his cardiologists, he had one implanted. It worked. Today, twelve years after that near-fatal heart attack, he lives a richly fulfilling life, encouraging other heart patients, and biking because he loves biking—not just to outrace the Angel of Death.

Don still "sings his heart out." Still plays his trumpet, too. But I don't think he's ever done *I Can't Stop Loving You* again!

♥ *Bonnie Compton Hanson*

# Get Off on the Right Foot . . . and Then the Left

Regular exercise can greatly reduce your risk of heart disease and help you rebound from a heart attack. Many doctors prescribe exercise in the form of cardiac rehabilitation for their heart patients because its effects are so powerful.

**Getting started:** You don't look good in sweats, you're not coordinated, you're out of shape . . . it's not difficult to come up with a hundred reasons not to exercise. The truth is, all you need to do is set aside a little time. Even ten minutes three times a week is a good start. Then work your way up to thirty minutes a day as your stamina improves. You don't even have to leave the house. You can exercise with a video in front of your TV in the privacy of your own home just as effectively as exercising outdoors or at the gym.

To get the most out of your exercise routine, try to work out with weights at least some of the time. Oh, you don't have weights? Fill empty plastic milk cartons with sand or water to a weight you can comfortably lift.

Good choices for working with weights include following an exercise video in your living room, joining an aerobics class with weights or even participating in yoga classes where you learn to flex your muscles and hold poses.

**How hard?** Make sure you're exercising hard enough to benefit your heart. Recommendation: Work out within your target heart rate zone. Find your zone this way:

Start with                       220
Subtract your age        _____
Multiply by .5               _____
Multiply by .75            _____ = target heart rate range

A fifty-year-old, for instance, would have a target heart rate range from 85 to 127 beats per minute (220 − 50 = 170 x .5 and .75).

If you're just starting to exercise, aim for the lowest part of the zone and then gradually build up to the higher part of the zone. You never want to exercise at your maximum heart rate range.

Take the talk test: If you can talk to an exercise partner or walking buddy, you're probably exercising hard enough. If you can't talk and feel as if you're exhausted, you're exercising too hard.

**How often?** Do activities that get your heart pumping at this rate for at least twenty minutes four times per week, or thirty minutes three times per week. But also look at what you're doing the rest of the day. Don't take the easy way, such as the escalator or elevator; take the stairs to add activity into your daily tasks. Park at the far end of a parking lot. Deliver messages in person instead of phoning. Walk the length of the shopping mall a few times, even if you're there just to stop at one store.

**How to find your heart rate:** Place your index or middle finger (not your thumb) just to the side of your Adam's apple on your neck, where you can feel your heartbeat. You may also try placing both fingers on the inside of your wrist (this takes some practice). Count the number of heartbeats for ten seconds and multiply by six (or count for six seconds and multiply by ten). That's your heart rate.

## Get Up, Get Moving

You have a "heart condition," so any exercise needs to be cleared by your doctor first. Even when your doctor gives you the green light, it is probably safer to exercise at a hospital-sponsored wellness center where trained staff can keep a close eye on you, and rescue personnel and equipment are right on site.

- **Walking** is a great way to get started, especially if you haven't exercised before or as you're transitioning from cardiac rehab where walking was a routine part of your workout. If you're concerned that walking will put stress on your back, hips or knees, you may want to try walking in a swimming pool.

- **Cycling**, either on a real bicycle or on a stationary machine, provides a good aerobic workout. For best results try riding up and down gentle hills. Be sure you dial up at least some resistance on stationary machines.
- **Aerobic dance** is a great way to get fit and meet new people. Many aerobic classes incorporate weight training into their routines. Low-impact aerobics, in which one foot is always on the ground (no jumping or running in place), is safer, especially if you're new to exercise or more than a little bit overweight.
- **Swimming** exercises your whole body and won't overstress your muscles and joints. Pushing the water away from you provides natural resistance that builds up your muscles. You can add to the resistance effect by using handheld paddles.
- **Circuit training** with weight machines is a highly effective technique available in most gyms. Hire a personal trainer for just a few sessions so you can learn proper technique and appropriate weight ranges.

♥ *Think about . . .*
## which exercise is right for me?

My favorite activities are:

\_\_ Aerobics

\_\_ Basketball

\_\_ Bicycling

\_\_ Dancing

\_\_ Golf

\_\_ Hiking

\_\_ Jogging

\_\_ Soccer

\_\_ Swimming

\_\_ Tennis

\_\_ Walking

\_\_ Weights

\_\_ Yoga

\_\_ Other: _____

_____

My favorite exercise is_____.

My goal is to do it _____ times a week for _____ minutes.

## Ancient Alternative: Tai Chi

Tai chi is a traditional Chinese martial art that has been practiced in China for centuries. Tai chi combines deep breathing with relaxation and postures that flow from one to another through slow movements. Tai chi is practiced to promote good health, memory, concentration, digestion, balance and flexibility and is thought to improve anxiety and depression.

Researchers found benefits in this ancient practice for people who had undergone heart bypass surgery, had high blood pressure and various types of heart conditions—and for healthy people, too.

- ♥ **Why does tai chi work?** Ah, that is the ancient question that has no answer.

- ♥ **Where can you find tai chi classes?** Check your local fitness or yoga center. Sometimes classes are offered by university recreation departments. Some personal instructors may provide one-on-one classes.

♥

## Serious as a Heart Attack

*A happy heart is better than a full purse.*

—ITALIAN PROVERB

I'm forty, from the Deep South and have a frightening family health history. The main cause, I suspect, is a historic diet of Southern-fried and pickled cuisine. To put a few minor health fears to rest (at my wife's urging), I agreed to get some tests. The last test, a coronary baseline, would be my ticket to a clean bill of health.

I had a morning appointment. The nurse stuck electrode patches all over me, snapping wires to each one. When she'd finished I looked like an extra from a sci-fi movie. The doctor walked in just as she finished, announcing, "It's time for the pain to begin!"

Running on a treadmill—not walking or jogging, but running—was a new experience for me. As I raced toward the blank white wall, sweat flowing from every pore, my thoughts were split between (a) the possible consequences of tripping while running on a treadmill, and (b) could I, through some freak miscalculation of moisture/electricity, be electrocuted by all these wires?

The test equipment, which looks suspiciously like

the engine diagnostic machine at the Ford dealership, beeped and chirped as the doctor studied the display. When the test was over, the doctor's demeanor changed. I recognized the same look mechanics have given me a hundred times, "Payday!"

"It's probably nothing, Banjo," he said calmly, "but you test positive for heart disease."

Stifling a gasp, I swallowed audibly, "How much time have I got, Steve?" All doctor/patient protocol went out the window with those three little words "It's probably nothing," the unluckiest phrase ever uttered by a doctor. Don't they understand? *Nothing*'s the deadliest disease known to Hollywood!

"No, you're not dying," Steve said, licking his lips as he calculated the fees he'd soon generate, "but we need to run additional tests. I'd like to bring in a cardiologist to examine you, but it's probably just a glitch, happens all the time."

I didn't worry my wife, Bonne, with the gory details that night. I just glazed over it, telling her there'd be more tests, but I was fine.

The next day I awoke with a stabbing pain in my left shoulder. I attributed it to my treadmill "fun run" and went to work. As the day progressed, so did the pain, into my chest and down my arm. I couldn't breathe without pain, and I was sweating. *Maybe I pinched a nerve,* I thought, *or . . . I'm having a heart attack!*

I called Steve. He was out on his yacht named *It's Probably Nothing,* so I described my condition to another doctor.

"Mr. Bandolas, I'm looking at yesterday's test," she said. "Did your doctor tell you it's positive for heart disease?"

*Why does everyone keep asking me that?* I wondered, assuring her I knew. "But he said it was a glitch?!?"

"Hmmmmmm."

An hour later I'd been checked into Sacred Heart Hospital's Cardiac Unit. The nurses took away my dignity and left me with a gown that, well, I guess everything needs to be accessible. The cardiologist arrived. We went over my symptoms again as he probed and prodded me.

"Did you know you test positive for heart disease?"

"I'm dying, aren't I?"

"We'll run some tests to be sure, but your pain doesn't seem to be heart-related."

An orderly arrived with a wheelchair. He got me some hospital pants (funny, the nurses never mentioned pants), and wheeled me to the torture, I mean, testing area. Way down in sublevel four where no one can hear you scream.

They wired me up again. Between attaching and ripping off electrodes, I barely had a strand of chest hair left. This time they added a new twist to the treadmill test: run until ready to plant face into hurtling treadmill belt. Leap, gracefully as a three-legged gazelle, onto a cold metal table. *Now the hard part.* Stop gasping like a stranded goldfish, assume the most painful contortion possible and hold your breath as they inspect your heart with the echocardiogram.

The echocardiogram shows a picture, like the sonogram used to inspect developing babies. So as I lay there, wincing and turning blue, I saw *INSIDE* my heart. I should have been fascinated.

The short of it, if that's possible at this point, is I'm just fine. It *was* just a glitch. I had a minor case of pleurisy. But it opened my eyes. So I'm taking steps. Literally taking steps. I walk and take the stairs as much as possible. I've also made some painful choices about food. The junk food, hamburgers and deliciously greasy burritos are gone. I'm healthy, and I can never take that for granted again.

♥ *Banjo Bandolas*

# DASH—Your Heart-Healthy Eating Plan

DASH stands for Dietary Approaches to Stop Hypertension, which is, of course, high blood pressure. This eating plan (note they don't call it a diet) can lower your blood pressure within two weeks. So make the dash to the DASH eating plan (developed by the National Heart, Lung and Blood Institute) to lower your blood pressure.

It's easy to adopt the DASH eating plan. Here are some ways to get started:

**Change gradually.**

- If you now eat one or two vegetables a day, add a serving at lunch and another at dinner.
- If you don't eat fruit now or have only juice at breakfast, add a serving to your meals or have it as a snack.
- Use only half the butter, margarine or salad dressing you do now.
- Try low-fat or fat-free condiments, such as fat-free salad dressings.
- Gradually increase dairy products to three servings per day. For example, drink milk with lunch or dinner instead of soda, alcohol or sugar-sweetened tea. Choose low-fat (1 percent) or fat-free (skim) dairy products to reduce total fat intake.

**Treat meat as one part of the whole meal, instead of the focus.**

- Buy less meat. If it's not there, you won't eat it.
- Limit meat to six ounces a day (two servings). Three to four ounces is about the size of a deck of cards.
- If you now eat large portions of meat, cut back gradually by a half or a third at each meal.
- Include two or more vegetarian-style (meatless) meals each week.
- Increase servings of vegetables, rice, pasta and dry beans in meals. Try casseroles, pasta and stir-fry dishes that have less meat and more vegetables, grains and dry beans.

**Use fruits or low-fat foods as desserts and snacks.**

- Fruits and low-fat foods offer great taste and variety. Use fruits canned in their own juice. Fresh fruits require little or no preparation. Dried fruits are easy to carry with you.
- Try these snack ideas: unsalted pretzels or nuts mixed with raisins; graham crackers; low-fat and fat-free yogurt and frozen yogurt; plain popcorn with no salt or butter added; raw vegetables.

## The DASH Eating Plan

The DASH eating plan is based on *2,000 calories a day*. The number of daily servings in a food group may vary from those listed depending on your caloric needs.

| Food Group | Daily Servings (except as noted) | Serving Sizes |
| --- | --- | --- |
| Grains and grain | 7–8 | 1 slice bread<br>1 cup ready-to-eat cereal*<br>½ cup cooked rice, pasta or cereal products |
| Vegetables | 4–5 | 1 cup raw leafy vegetable<br>½ cup cooked vegetable<br>6 ounces vegetable juice |
| Fruits | 4–5 | 1 medium fruit<br>½ cup dried fruit<br>½ cup fresh, frozen or canned fruit<br>6 ounces fruit juice |
| Low-fat or fat-free dairy foods | 2–3 | 8 ounces milk<br>1 cup yogurt<br>1½ ounces cheese |
| Lean meats, poultry and fish | 2 or less | 3 ounces cooked lean meats, skinless poultry or fish |
| Nuts, seeds and dry beans | 4–5 per week | ⅓ cup or 1½ ounces nuts<br>1 tablespoon or ½ ounce seeds<br>½ cup cooked dry beans |

* Serving sizes vary between ½ cup–1¼ cups. Check the product's nutrition label.

| Food Group | Daily Servings (except as noted) | Serving Sizes |
| --- | --- | --- |
| Fats and oils** | 2–3 | 1 teaspoon soft margarine<br>1 tablespon low-fat mayonnaise<br>2 tablespoons light salad dressing<br>1 teaspoon vegetable oil |
| Sweets | 5 per week | 1 tablespoon sugar<br>1 tablespoon jelly or jam<br>½ ounce jelly beans<br>8 ounces lemonade |

** Fat content changes serving counts for fats and oils: For example, 1 tablespoon of regular salad dressing equals 1 serving; 1 tablespoon of a low-fat dressing equals ½ serving; 1 tablespoon of a fat-free dressing equals 0 servings.

# Tips on How to Make
# Heart-Healthier Meals

**Begin by choosing foods low in saturated fat, low in sodium and low in calories:**

- Try fat-free (skim) milk or low-fat (1 percent) milk.
- Only buy cheeses marked "low-fat" or "fat-free" on the package.
- Choose to eat fruits and vegetables without butter or sauce.
- Serve rice, beans, cereals, pasta and whole grains (such as couscous, barley and bulgur).
- Choose lean cuts of meat, fish and skinless turkey and chicken.
- When available, buy low- or reduced-sodium or no-salt-added versions of foods.

**Use these recipe substitutions:**

- Use two egg whites for each whole egg and margarine or oil instead of butter.
- Use light mayonnaise instead of the regular variety.
- Use nonfat yogurt instead of sour cream.
- Use low-fat cheese instead of regular cheese.
- Use 1 percent or skim milk instead of whole milk.

- Use fresh poultry, fish and lean meat rather than canned or processed types.

**Try these meal tips:**

- Make a meatloaf with lean ground turkey.
- Make tacos with skinless chicken breast.
- Cool soups and gravies, and skim off fat before reheating them.
- Try adding salsa on a baked potato instead of butter.
- Make a spicy baked fish—season with green pepper, onion, garlic, oregano, lemon or cilantro.
- Eat fruit for dessert, instead of pie or cake.

## Shake the Salt Habit

Salt (also called sodium on food labels) can raise blood pressure. That's why tight control on sodium in the DASH diet is vital for lowering dangerously high blood pressure. The average American consumes from 4,000 to 6,000 milligrams of sodium a day. You want to shoot for 1,500 milligrams a day. That's about 2/3 of a teaspoon of table salt.

It's not that you add this much salt to foods. Sodium is present in many foods such as frozen dinners and pizza, instant rice, canned soups and broth, salad dressing, and canned vegetables and tuna.

Shake the salt habit by removing the salt shaker from your table and don't reach for it without tasting food first. You can "unlearn" your taste for salt.

**Here's how:**

- Read the Nutrition Facts label for sodium content in a single serving. Track your sodium intake each day and try to stay under 1,500 mg.
- Drain and rinse canned foods, even tuna, vegetables and beans, to remove excess salt.
- Use spices instead of salt in cooking and at the table. Flavor foods with herbs, lemon, lime, vinegar and salt-free seasoning blends.
- Use fresh poultry, fish and lean meat rather than canned, smoked or processed.
- Cook rice, pasta and hot cereals without salt added to the water.

# My Page

My Thoughts _____

_____

_____

_____

My Feelings _____

_____

_____

_____

My Facts _____

_____

_____

_____

My Support _____

_____

_____

_____

♥

## Mission Possible: Healing One Heart from Baghdad

*The best and most beautiful things in the world cannot be seen or even touched. They must be felt within the heart.*

—Helen Keller

It had been an exhausting pilgrimage from their war-torn home in Baghdad to New York, but Najwa Mohammed was on a mission to save her four-year-old daughter's life. Bar`aa had been born with a complex congenital heart defect called Tetralogy of Fallot, which causes cyanosis, often called "blue baby." The combination of several abnormalities starved her body of oxygen, making her weak and causing her to pass out on several occasions.

She needed an operation to repair her heart, and Project Kids Worldwide, a nonprofit organization based at NYU Medical Center, had accepted the child for surgery and located a sponsor to underwrite the expenses because the war had left no hospitals equipped or surgeons capable of performing the complex heart surgery in Iraq.

As the representative from Project Kids Worldwide, I was accompanied by a diplomat from the Iraqi

Mission to the United Nations. We officially welcomed the mother and child at the airport in New York. Although Bar`aa was playful at the airport, her lips and fingernails were noticeably blue, an indicator that her condition was worsening.

We drove Najwa and Bar`aa to a home in the Bronx where a host family was awaiting their arrival. Joy and Alex Schtakleff and their three daughters had busied themselves preparing the room where Najwa and Bar`aa would stay. Shrills of excitement were heard throughout the house as the girls watched the car pull up. There were lots of hugs and kisses as Najwa and Bar`aa arrived at the Schtakleffs' home. They all seemed to sense that this might be the beginning of an experience that would unite their hearts forever.

On Sunday afternoon, a reporter interviewed Najwa regarding her amazing journey from Baghdad and Bar`aa's impending surgery. During the interview, a photo album on the dining-room table was opened to a picture of an astronaut standing on the moon's surface.

"Who is this?" I asked.

"My father," Joy replied. It was astronaut James B. Irwin of the *Apollo 15* crew—the eighth man to walk on the moon.

Soon after his historic space flight, Colonel Irwin wrote: "I felt very special when I looked down at my footprints on the moon. The scientists said they would be there for a million years. Looking up I could see the Earth the size of a marble. It was so beautiful and so far away. And yet I felt strangely at home on the moon."

Could our young Iraqi mother and her child, thousands of miles away from their native soil, somehow feel at home in New York, a place so remote from anything they had ever known? For them, it might as well have been the moon.

On Monday afternoon, Bar`aa was evaluated by NYU Medical Center's pediatric cardiology team, and her surgery was scheduled for Wednesday morning. Dr. Stephen B. Colvin, Chief of Cardiothoracic Surgery and cofounder of Project Kids Worldwide, would perform the operation. Bar`aa's little heart would be in the hands of one of the most highly skilled surgeons in the world.

On the morning of the surgery, a nurse came for Bar`aa and gave Najwa a blue sterile gown to cover her ash-colored burka. She would go with Bar`aa into the sterile operating room. As the anxious mother quietly carried her precious angel into the room, she was softly singing an Arabic prayer. Najwa tried to hold back her tears until Bar`aa was asleep. Her composure was testimony to her strength during the five-hour surgery.

When Najwa was allowed to go into the recovery

room, she began to cry. Dr. Colvin was at the child's bedside reassuring the mother that the surgery had been a complete success. International media covering the surgery sent the story around the world with a simple message: One little Iraqi girl had received the gift of life as so many other lives were being lost in the war.

When asked how he felt, Dr. Colvin remarked to one reporter, "I am very fortunate to be able to take care of patients and perform complex surgery." And like another pioneer whose footprints remain on the moon, Dr. Colvin, too, felt a deep sense of accomplishment when he said, "I feel like this is part of my mission."

Stepping into the unknown takes courage. Whether performing surgery inside the delicate chambers of the heart, exploring the surface of the moon or traveling to a foreign land to save a child's life, we are each called to missions in our lives. Some may seem to be impossible. But the footprints we leave behind will be remembered. Some for a lifetime. Some for a million years.

♥ *Deborah D. Coble*
Project Kids Worldwide

# What's My Alternative?

Meditation, yoga, prayerful reflection, music therapy and your own furry family dog Fido could all be thought of as complementary medicine.

Complementary medicine, or integrative medicine, combines mainstream medical therapies (such as surgery for heart disease or medicine for high blood pressure) with alternative practices that have proven safety and effectiveness.

Be sure to discuss with your doctor any complementary practices you undertake. Why? Because certain herbs (a form of alternative medicine) may interact with medications you might be taking to control blood pressure and cholesterol or to thin your blood in preventing stroke. But noninvasive practices such as meditation or yoga may indeed heighten the effects of your recovery and prevention efforts, and your doctor may be very supportive.

Some helpful complementary practices:

- **Meditation:** Scientists are not quite certain how meditation works, but perhaps we can gain some insight from the work of Harvard's Herbert Benson, M.D., who initially wrote about the relaxation response. Images in your head of a quiet stream or a flower-laden forest can lower blood pressure, lower pulse and have tremendous benefits if you have heart disease. Picturing serenity, achieving bliss in your mind's eye—this is the very basis of human pursuits. Through mental imagery and other meditation techniques, prayer and other types of cerebral activities, you can fight against disease. Whether or not these techniques prolong life is unclear, but they certainly enhance the quality of life and empower you in this most difficult of all of life's journeys.

- **Pets:** When you stroke your pet, within minutes your brain releases a spa treatment of brain chemicals that makes you feel good—and your pet receives similar benefits, too. "Heavy petting" creates a sensory reaction similar to what takes place when a mother nurses her baby. This type of therapeutic touch really works to provide relaxation.

  Petting pets lowers blood pressure. Perhaps that's why pet owners take less medication for high blood pressure and high cholesterol. This puts pet owners at a reduced risk for heart disease. Even among people who suffered heart attacks, pet owners had a four times better chance of surviving one year than did those who did not have pets. Pets also keep you moving. Sometimes your best exercise partner is your dog. And pets can buffer your reaction to acute stress. A few minutes alone with your cat or dog might do more to help your stress than talking about your troubles with a best (human) friend or spouse.

- **Laughter:** Health and healing are laughing matters, really. If you're looking forward to a favorite comedy on TV, just checking the TV listings may trigger healthy mood changes, reduce your stress hormone levels and boost your immune system's defenses. Even anticipating a laugh-inducing event reduces levels of tension, anger, depression, fatigue and confusion up to two days *before* the actual event. Why? Because your brain releases a cascade of feel-good hormones that provide a "runner's high"—a feeling of wellness—and boost your immune system. Laughter and humor are free medicine. Take a dose every day.

## ♥ Think about . . .
## my complementary practices

Which of these practices can you add to your "treatment" plan?

__ Meditation

__ Mental Imagery

__ Yoga

__ Laughter

__ Pets

__ Music

__ Healing Touch

__ Prayer

__ Social Interaction

__ Volunteerism

__ Art

__ Tai chi

# How to Meditate

Mindful breathing and sitting (meditation) help to relax and focus the mind. Just five minutes a day can make you feel more refreshed and energetic. Here are some guidelines for practicing mindful breathing and sitting:

- ♥ Make a special time and place for "nondoing."

- ♥ Adopt an alert and relaxed body posture.

- ♥ Look dispassionately at the reactions and habits of your mind.

- ♥ Bring your attention to your breathing by counting silently "1" on inhalation and "2" on exhalation, "3" on inhalation, and so on. When you reach number "10," return to number "1." (If you go beyond the number 10, then you know your mind has wandered.) When your mind wanders, name what it wanders to and come back to the breathing.

Reprinted by permission of the Women's Heart Foundation.

♥

## In a Heartbeat

*Sometimes the heart sees*
*what is invisible to the eye.*

—U<small>NKNOWN</small>

I had had a very long day and night "on call," finally crawling into my call-room bed well after midnight. A shrill page jerked me awake.

"**Anesthesia.** STAT to ER! Anesthesia. **STAT** to ER!"

As a certified registered nurse anesthetist (CRNA), I not only provide anesthesia for surgery, but am also called when hearts or breathing have stopped.

I shoved my feet into my shoes and hit the door running. In seconds, I was pushing my way into the emergency room. It looked like a madhouse or maybe a firefighter convention as I pushed past men clad in yellow gear to reach the patient.

The soot-blackened face on the stretcher looked about thirty. Not breathing. Full cardiac arrest. Distantly I heard the information offered by the firefighters as I illuminated his airway and slipped a tube into his trachea. Life-giving oxygen filled his lungs, replacing his absent breath.

They'd fought a chemical warehouse fire. He

was inside. He'd seemed okay when the fire was contained, but unusually quiet afterward. Tired, he said. Just stripping out of his gear when he collapsed. Unresponsive on arrival to the ER.

We followed cardiac protocol though a diagnosis wasn't clear. Heart attack? Smoke inhalation? Chemical poisoning?

I breathed for him in-between chest compressions in the dance of modern CPR. Cardiac drugs into the IV. Look for effect. Shouts of "Clear!" Defibrillate to restore normal rhythm. Minutes ticked by. He'd been down thirty minutes. Then forty-five.

"Pause CPR." Check the monitor. "Resume CPR." With each report, we saw no signs our fervent ministrations were working.

And then I heard it. The men who braved danger together, standing as a band of brothers, began to call his name. At first, they'd stepped back, professionals allowing us to do our job. But now they surrounded the stretcher, standing behind those working to save their friend. Still stained with soot, they rallied their comrade.

"Come on, Joe! Don't give up!"

"We love ya, Man!"

"We're here, Buddy! Hang in there!"

"Come on, Joe! Don't leave us, Buddy!"

With outstretched arms, they pleaded for their

colleague to come back to them from wherever he had gone. Tears fell unchecked as deep voices cracked with emotion. Our clinical discussion was silenced by the life-and-death tug-of-war they fought for their friend. We did not speak what we were thinking, *We've done everything! There is nothing more to do,* until finally the doctor broke our silence.

"One last time. Stop CPR. Check the monitor."

I continued gently inflating the lungs of the man I now knew as Joe. The doctor would decide when to stop. I watched the monitor.

One blip. Then another. And then one complex after another marching across the screen in normal sinus rhythm.

"Check for a pulse!" The doctor's voice held a quiver of excitement.

I felt his neck. "I have a pulse!"

The ER cheered, firefighters and staff alike. We knew we had seen a miracle. A massive heart attack was the final diagnosis, but Joe recovered easily, soon going home to his wife and kids.

I would like to say it was the miracle of modern medicine that saved Joe, but I know in my heart that, instead, it was that oldest of cures: the love of friends who wouldn't give up combined with the tenacious will of the human spirit to live.

❤ *Kimberly Zweygardt*

# Classic Signs of Heart Attack

It never happens like in the movies. Heart attack can sneak up on you, strike at the most inopportune moment, to some of the most surprisingly healthy people. Your best defense is knowledge about what to look for. Take these signs seriously:

- **Sudden, intense pressure** (as if an elephant were sitting on your chest), squeezing, fullness, tightness, burning or pain in the chest that lasts more than a few minutes
- **Chest pain** that travels to the arm, neck, jaw, inside arm, shoulder (left side more than right), upper abdomen (often mistaken for indigestion pain) or back between the shoulder blades—pain may be continuous or come and go
- **Chest discomfort** and feeling lightheaded
- **Shortness of breath,** dizziness
- **Fainting**
- **Sweating,** clamminess
- **Nausea**
- **Vomiting**

These classic signs apply more commonly to men. Here are the more unlikely but potentially deadly symptoms that a woman should not ignore:

- Unexplained exhaustion, fatigue, weakness
- Unexplained shortness of breath
- Chest discomfort: pressure, tingling, squeezing, full feeling
- Full feeling in neck, discomfort in jaw, ear, teeth with exertion
- Stomach distress (feeling as if you could just belch)
- Discomfort in upper shoulder blades in back
- Discomfort in one or both arms
- Unexplained nausea/dizziness
- Heart palpitations (feeling your heart beat), cold sweat

## Classic Signs of Stroke

Much like a heart attack, a stroke is a "brain attack" in which blood vessels in the brain or leading to the brain are blocked by a blood clot, or a blood vessel in the brain has burst.

Signs and symptoms of stroke:

- **Sudden weakness** or **numbness** of the face, arm or leg on one side of the body
- **Sudden dimness** or loss of vision, particularly in one eye
- **Sudden confusion**, or trouble talking or understanding speech
- **Sudden, severe headache** with no known or apparent cause

- **Unexplained dizziness,** unsteadiness or sudden falls, especially along with any of the other symptoms

**Ministrokes** (known as transient ischemic attacks or TIAs) occur when the blood supply is temporarily cut off by a clot in the brain. TIA and stroke symptoms can be the same, but a TIA is temporary and may last only a few minutes. This is a warning sign that a major stroke is about to occur. Seek immediate medical attention.

### Take One Minute, Ask Three Simple Questions

Mom suddenly starts to slur her speech. Dad's arm goes numb. One side of a coworker's face droops. These are signs of stroke, and quick thinking may speed life-saving treatment.

You may be able to spot someone having a stroke by taking one minute and asking three simple questions:

1. **Can you smile?** A droopy smile to one side can indicate paralysis, a sign of a stroke.
2. **Can you raise both arms over your head?** Arm weakness is a sign of a stroke.
3. **Can you talk to me?** Slurry speech is one more sign of stroke.

♥

## A Shocking Start

*If it were not for hope, the heart would break.*
*He who has health has hope;*
*and he who has hope has everything.*

—Thomas Fuller

"Security. This is Ford Hudson," I said, answering the phone at the security gate of the engineering facility for International Truck and Engine in Fort Wayne, Indiana.

"Tom Crandall collapsed. It's an emergency," said the caller. When the call for help came in from a colleague at the desk next to Tom's, I grabbed the automated external defibrillator (AED) and the first-aid kit. You never know what the circumstances might be.

It took me less than a minute to reach Tom's cubicle in a large work area. When I got to Tom's desk, I found him slumped back in his chair. "Tom. Hey, Tom. Can you hear me?" No response. His arms were rigidly locked under the arms of his desk chair. He was purple.

I wasn't sure how much time had elapsed, but my first-responder training for my job as a security guard kicked into overdrive. I radioed more guards for assistance.

I knew I had to get Tom lying flat on the floor quickly, but I had trouble getting him out of the chair because his arms were jammed so tightly. Get to the chest. I wasn't even thinking, just doing. I ripped open his shirt. I checked for a pulse. Nothing. I checked for breath. None. It was the worst-case scenario.

This isn't something we guards do on a regular basis, so the adrenalin started pumping and our training kicked in. Fortunately, I had just been recertified in CPR and AED two days earlier. The AED is a suitcase-sized device that delivers life-saving shock to restore normal rhythm in an irregularly beating heart. Or shocks the heart into beating if the heart isn't beating at all.

"No pulse," I called out to the two guards who came to my assistance. "We're going to need the AED."

I flipped open the case, got out the two pads and placed them on Tom's chest where we were trained to put them. A diagram on the case also showed me that I had them aligned just right.

The machine assesses the victim and gives a "shock" or "no shock" signal.

The "shock" indicator lit up. "Stand clear," I announced, "we're gonna shock," and then I pushed the button.

We waited. The machine analyzed the signal

from Tom's heart once again. His heart must have been quivering, but not beating. The machine signaled me, "Shock." I pushed the button again.

We held our breath. And again the "shock" signal flashed. Another and another.

The paramedics rushed in. I told them we had delivered four shocks. They hooked Tom up to their more sophisticated equipment and delivered two more powerful shocks to jump-start our friend.

Still no response. We were sure he was gone.

*I woke up five days later in the hospital with three new stents in place in my coronary arteries. My cardiologist calls me his "miracle." Most people aren't lucky enough to have a cardiac arrest near an AED and people trained to deliver the lifesaving shock. It took this life event for me to finally quit smoking. Yes, I got the message, and I was back at work in a month.*

*What do you say to a guy who saves your life? It's tough. I didn't remember a thing after the conference call. My lifesavers filled in the details. When Ford mentioned they ripped off my shirt, I kidded him, "You owe me a shirt."*

*Home heart monitoring showed that my irregular heartbeat could cause problems again, so a few months later doctors implanted a pacemaker in my chest, equipped to deliver a shock to regulate my heart. I've never felt it, but I'm told if the device kicks in, the shock will feel as if I had put my finger in a light socket.*

*The mayor honored the three guards who aided me, including Ford, with commendations for heroism. Ford claims the machine saved my life. I know his quick action and training really made it happen.*

*I retired a few months after the incident. Even though I didn't want a retirement party, the office organized a little coffee and cake. A few people said nice things about me, then Ford got up.*

*"Tom, we got this little gift for you. For your retirement." I opened the box. It was a shirt.*

*"I guess this makes us even now," I said in deep appreciation for much more than a shirt.*

*♥ Ford Hudson and Thomas Crandall*

# Six Minutes to Save a Life

If someone you're with . . .

- Faints or collapses suddenly
- Stops breathing
- Has no pulse
- Has twitching muscles

. . . you have just six minutes to save a life.

What to do in the chain of survival:

1. Call 9-1-1 emergency services right away.
2. Give CPR because compressing the person's chest keeps blood flowing to the brain and the rest of the body.
3. Ask a bystander to find out if there is a nearby automated external defibrillator—an instrument used to shock the heart out of its deadly pace and back into a normal, steady rhythm.

Fast emergency care can make the difference between life and death.

# When Is a Heart Attack a 9-1-1 Emergency?

Trick question. Heart attack is **always** an emergency, but most people having heart attacks don't think so. Especially younger people. Nearly half of heart-attack patients drive themselves or were driven to the hospital.

Here are three smart reasons to call for an ambulance:

1. You are more likely to be taken to the best cardiac centers.
2. Half of heart-attack patients die within the first hour.
3. Paramedics begin treatment right away and will alert the hospital in advance with critical data.

In the few minutes you're waiting for the squad, chew an aspirin. Chewing gets the blood-thinning effects into your system immediately. Tell the paramedics you have taken an aspirin.

## ♥ *Think about . . .*
## my emergency plan

Having a heart attack increases your chances of having another one. Talk to your doctor and your family about making an **emergency action plan.**

**My emergency action plan:**

The signs and symptoms of a heart attack are:

_____

_____

_____

My doctor's instructions for the prompt use of aspirin and nitroglycerin are:

_____

How many? _____

How often? _____

When to call the doctor? _____

The location of the nearest hospital that offers twenty-four-hour emergency heart care is:

_____

♥

## Thanks for the Miracle, Sis

*"Hope" is the thing with feathers—*
*That perches in the soul—*
*And sings the tune without the words—*
*And never stops—at all—*

—EMILY DICKINSON

My Dear Sister Sally,

When I left you at the rehab center after your second stroke at age forty-six, you were paralyzed on your left side, confined to bed, confused about what was happening. Doctors said you could die, or at best subsist with extensive brain damage. Yet eight weeks later, you greet me at the airport— leaning on your cane, your hair freshly styled, tears running down your face.

I came to check on you, but you taught me.

Sure, you still have weakness in your left arm and don't always immediately process what's said. You mispronounce some words and grow confused if we talk too fast, but *you* are intact: your keen intelligence, your delicious sense of humor, your thoughtfulness and generosity, your sweet soul. More folks should be as whole as you are.

Thank you for your example in courage,

fortitude and persistence in the face of great odds.

I saw you punch numbers into the automatic teller machine to get your bank balance, then do it all again when you forgot the sum. And I was suddenly ashamed that some days simply getting out of bed seems like too much work for me.

Thank you for your laughter. When you go for your weekly blood draws to see if your blood thinner's working, you're off to "the vampire's." When you looked at the bleak hospital photos I'd snapped of you attached to snakelike tubes, you quipped, "I was really having a bad hair day!" Boy, are you a lesson in lightening up.

Several times you apologized "for being trouble." Don't you know how grateful we are, dear Sally, to finally be able to give back to you? Who else but you would hand out Christmas gifts in January—gifts you'd purchased long before the stroke, now wrapped in paper bags because you couldn't manage gift-wrapping?

Thank you for pointing out what's truly important—and for saying that you'd dropped from your list nagging your teenager about his room. "I used to worry about things I thought were problems—like being fat," you said. "Heavy isn't a problem. Being healthy is the most important thing in the world." Let me remember that the next time I climb onto the scale.

And thanks, too, for the lesson in gentleness with yourself. When you pulled your shirt on inside-out and we pointed it out, you didn't beat yourself up as we so often do over mistakes. You simply said, "Oops, I flunked shirt!" and fixed it. And when you said to your sisters, "I'm so glad I didn't die. I woulda missed you guys."

We would have missed you, too, Sal. My miracle sister.

♥ *Jann Mitchell*

♥ *Think about . . .*
living day to day

Caregivers can often become so involved in the day-to-day efforts to keep things going, they tend to forget that each day can be an opportunity to try new approaches and activities that will make a positive difference in their life and in the lives of those they care for.

If you're a caregiver, stand back and take a look at your situation: What is working well, and what isn't? How can you find ways to make changes for the better?

Ideas that may be helpful:

♥ What can you use to make life easier?

— Communication devices such as a cordless speaker phone, a cell phone, one-touch dialing for emergencies, an intercom system to use when you are in another room, or a medical alert necklace that, when activated, calls emergency services

— Assistive devices such as special eating utensils for stroke patients, plastic chair for the shower, a wheelchair for use in situations that require a lot of walking (airports, shopping malls, grocery stores)

— A handicapped parking permit to allow closer parking

— A notebook that contains lists of medications and emergency contacts (names and phone numbers for family members, doctors, pharmacy, physical therapy, cardiac rehab, home health agency, wellness center) so you as caregiver can turn over the helm and have all vital information at hand for someone filling in as caregiver (and for emergency medical services)

— A binder that contains all medical records for easy reference and tracking of cholesterol, blood pressure, weight and other tests

♥ How can you support a heart patient making vital, lifesaving changes?

— Plan activities you both like to do and look forward to, such as going to cardiac rehab and then enjoying a cup of coffee afterward

— Attend heart-healthy cooking classes to learn new recipes and methods of cooking (and eating)

— Invite others for meals (especially friends who will bring in a healthful meal)

— Rent exercise and activity videos—also movies and books on tape

— Be active together in community walks and fund-raisers

— Try yoga classes and learn to meditate

— Learn new hobbies and crafts

— Volunteer at health fairs for local heart organizations and donor services

— Plan active day trips

— Consider a pet

# My Page

My Thoughts _____

_____

_____

_____

My Feelings _____

_____

_____

_____

My Facts _____

_____

_____

_____

My Support _____

_____

_____

_____

♥

## Cradled in God's Hands

*The human heart is like a ship on a stormy sea*
*driven about by winds blowing*
*from all four corners of heaven.*

—MARTIN LUTHER

It is midnight, and our kids and their spouses have all arrived from various cities and are catching up on the news. The past week has been hard. Every time I see the photograph on the mantle of my husband and me, the thought of losing him makes me want to die.

Early the next morning a somber group hovers around his bed as my husband is prepped for coronary bypass surgery. A male nurse in green garb says, "It's time to go."

The guys try to be macho and give him a high-five and "Hang in there, dude!" The girls kiss their father and hug him tight. I kiss him, maybe for the last time, and tears come to my eyes.

This six-foot man looks so small on the gurney in his blue-checkered gown. We wave as he is wheeled down the corridor until he is a speck in the distance. My husband is only fifty-four, but years of smoking, eating junk food and being a couch potato have taken their toll.

We set up camp in the waiting room, each bringing their own kind of security: magazines, water, apples and pillows. My two daughters decide to go to the hospital cafeteria and urge me to come along. I sit riveted to my chair, as if any movement will upset my facade of strength. I will the surgery to go well. I make deals with God. *If you let him live, I will never tell him to wear his jacket again. I won't nag him about taking out the trash. I will let him channel surf.*

As the hours stretch on, we all sit lost in our private thoughts and memories. My eldest daughter, seeing my pain, softly says, "Mom, just picture him cradled in God's hands. That's who's in charge now." I nod quietly. She's right. It is out of my hands.

Just when the wait seems unbearable, the nurse tells us to head for ICU. There are whoops of joy all around. He's not out of the woods, but doing well.

We are met with banks of monitors with their constant beeping, the "whoosh, whoosh" of the ventilator, and tubes of every size and description.

My son breaks down and has to leave the room. This father who never missed a Little League game or a drum-line competition looks so helpless now. The girls huddle together around the bed. I kiss my husband's cheek and rub his hand, the only place I can touch skin where there are no tubes.

The nurse says, "He is doing fine. He'll be groggy

all night; it would be better to come back tomorrow when he wakes up." She is right, and we agree to get some much-needed rest. We ride home in silence, feeling beat-up but relieved.

The next afternoon he is moved to a regular room. I see him for the first time without the tubes. He looks awful, but when he says, "Hi, babe," he is the most beautiful sight in the world.

In three days he is released from the hospital. In three weeks he enters cardiac rehab and actually learns to like exercise. Life changes. We cuddle more. He goes to the gym. I go back to work. Low-fat dinners become the norm. Luckily, he gave up smoking six months ago. One less hurdle.

In three months he is working full-time. We both learn to read food labels. Cholesterol, saturated fat, polyunsaturated fat, all foreign phrases a short time ago, are now in our everyday vocabulary. We're eating healthier and losing weight.

The culmination comes eight months later on a fall morning. My husband silently creeps out of bed early. He is gone a couple of hours. When he comes home he is wearing the biggest grin I have ever seen, and on his T-shirt is pinned the number 16. He has just run his first 5K. I finally exhale a long overdue sigh; life has begun anew.

♥ *Sallie Rodman*

# Cardiac Rehab: One Way to Save Your Life

Cardiac rehabilitation is a lifestyle program that includes medically supervised exercise to help people regain strength after a heart attack, bypass surgery, stroke or angioplasty. Even though exercise may be difficult for you, especially for older people, and even though exercise seems like the last thing you feel like doing, cardiac rehab can help you prevent another heart episode.

Follow your doctor's exercise prescription and show up at your supervised cardiac rehab sessions. These are usually held in a hospital setting or medically based wellness center under the guidance of cardiac nurses. You will wear a heart monitor and follow a set pattern of activity that might include walking on a treadmill, riding an exercise bike or simply walking around an inside track. All the while, your heart is being monitored remotely by the nurses.

You work up to more vigorous exercise until you finally graduate some weeks later. For patients who attended cardiac rehab, death rates in the following three-year period were the same as for people who had not had heart attacks. Cardiac rehab works so well, it's almost as if you never had a heart attack.

P.S.: The best way to boost your odds is to continue exercising on your own, once you graduate from cardiac rehab. Look for a cardiac rehab program that allows you to continue exercising at the same facility without the supervision. The transition—and the exercise habit you have built—will be easier to maintain. Plus, you'll already have plenty of friendly exercise partners and staff to cheer you on.

## More Than the Blues

Not bouncing back from your heart attack? Concerned about your progress in recovering from stroke?

After a heart attack, many people worry about having another heart attack. They often feel depressed and may have trouble adjusting to a new lifestyle.

If you're depressed, you are more than twice as likely to require bypass surgery, suffer other heart-related complications and have another heart attack.

Depression affects heart health. And it's not unusual for someone who has had a brush with death to feel depressed. The bad news is that you may not recognize your own depression. The good news is that depression can be cured.

Check the statements that apply to you. If you check five or more, and if these statements have been true for the past two weeks, you may have clinical depression. Your heart and your health will improve once you seek help from your doctor.

____ I feel sad, empty. Life seems hopeless.

____ I don't enjoy hobbies or activities that I used to.

____ Nothing brings me pleasure. Nothing matters.

____ I'm not hungry. Nothing sounds good, not even my favorite foods. And I am losing weight.

____ I can't stop eating, and my weight is climbing.

____ I can't get to sleep. Or, I can't sleep through the night. I keep waking up. Or, I seem to sleep all the time.

____ Every little thing makes me jump. I'm nervous all the time. I get startled easily.

____ I feel as if I'm plodding through the desert every day. Each step is difficult. I don't have as much energy as I used to.

____ Nothing I do is worthwhile. I just can't cut it.

____ I just can't think clearly. I keep forgetting things or I lose track. No way could I make a decision.

____ Maybe life just isn't worth living.

♥ *Think about . . .*
### ways to prevent (another) heart attack

1. **Make lifestyle changes.** Stop smoking. Learn to reduce stress. Exercise.

2. **Lower and control your blood pressure.** Try diet and exercise first to lower your blood pressure under 120/80. Your next strategy is to talk with your doctor about effective blood-pressure medications. Just because you may "feel better," don't stop taking these medicines on your own.

3. **Lower and control your cholesterol.** Lowering your cholesterol by forty total points reduces your heart attack risk by half. Drop another forty points, and your risk is cut in half again.

4. **Manage your weight.** A heart-healthy diet is the key to reducing your heart risk if you are overweight. Know your target weight and enlist the help of a registered dietitian.

5. **Take needed medications.** Know what you're taking and why, when to take it regularly and follow a plan.

# Is Taking a Daily Aspirin Right for You?

Taking a daily low-dose aspirin (81 to 160 milligrams) has been linked to a significantly lower risk of first heart attack, as well as protection against a second heart attack. An anti-inflammatory and blood thinner, aspirin reacts against chemicals that cause fever, swelling and pain in the body.

Some people are advised to stop taking aspirin before surgery or a procedure such as a colonoscopy. But once you start, don't stop taking aspirin without talking with your doctor first. And if you take other pain relievers such as ibuprofen for arthritis, take the aspirin a few hours before so they don't lessen the effects of each other.

Only you and your doctor can decide if taking a daily aspirin is right for you. Risks may include bleeding and complications from allergies to aspirin, but many experts think the benefits outweigh the risks, especially if you are at high risk for heart disease.

Also helpful:

- ♥ **Smile.** A smile a day keeps heart disease away. Do you look at life and see the glass half full or half empty? A sense of optimism may protect your health. Pessimism, on the other hand, may be linked to poor health.
- ♥ **Sex.** Men and women who had sexual intercourse most often (but nobody defined "how often") seemed to have fewer heart problems and lower death rates.
- ♥ **Fido.** Owning a dog, and actually walking the dog, leads to lowering risk for heart attack.

♥

## A Damaged Heart Finds Love

My internal physician, Dr. Leo, was absent. I visited one of his partners. "I'm tired and achy. And it feels cold inside my chest."

Putting his stethoscope against me, he said, "Have you been coughing up any mucus?"

"A little."

"Your chest sounds clear."

"I think it's my heart."

"Your heart? Let's not jump to extremes."

But Dr. Leo had once told me that aching could signify an infection of my replaced mitral valve, and it was nine years since my bicycle accident—a Ford Ranger truck had actually run over me. My heart surgeon, Dr. McConnell, had warned that the pig valve he'd used to replace my ripped mitral valve wouldn't last more than ten years. By age thirty-three, he'd said, I'd have to have a mechanical valve. I was thirty-two.

My cardiologist, Dr. Waider, had told me to have an echogram done yearly, but I was slacking and hadn't seen him for two. Now I was scared. I insisted to Dr. Leo's partner that I was sick. Handing me a prescription, he said, "Take these antibiotics for bronchitis for ten days."

Ten days later, I felt worse. I called another

partner of Dr. Leo. He prescribed more antibiotics. A few days later, I quit taking them and saw Dr. Waider.

"Your valve looks great."

"But why am I so achy?"

I left the office and sat in my car. "God," I prayed, "please let Dr. Leo be there." Without making an appointment, I drove to his office.

"He's just about to leave," the receptionist said. "But, I'll tell him you're here . . ."

As the receptionist was finishing her words, Dr. Leo appeared. I sighed. "Something's wrong," I said.

He led me into the examining room. "Let's draw some blood and do some tests. I'll call you tomorrow with the results."

I returned to my one-bedroom apartment and dropped onto my bed. My heart was racing.

The phone rang. "Hi, Greg," I said to my best friend for the last two years. I told him that I was worried about my heart.

"Call 911," he replied. After coughing up some blood, I did.

I was admitted to Long Beach Memorial Hospital. After performing another echogram, Dr. Waider explained that the antibiotics had masked my infected pig valve. Now I was in the Intensive Care Unit, on intravenous antibiotics. The diuretic that I was receiving was clearing up the fluid in my lungs.

As I lay with my eyes closed and my heart racing (literally), I heard a whistling that sounded like *woo-hoo, woo-hoo*. Then, I heard the nurses laughing. I opened my eyes to see my best friend nearing, holding a wicker basket of purple (my favorite color) flowers, with a whistling stuffed monkey hanging from a branch.

Greg explained how movement or noise prompted the monkey to whistle. "And since you can't have real flowers in ICU," he said, "I got you these fake ones."

Greg visited me nearly every day, and kept me smiling and laughing. While he was away, I thought of the time he had asked me to marry him. Although I had said no, he had remained a faithful friend.

A week later my infection cleared, and it was time to receive the mechanical valve. Just before surgery, while I lay on the gurney, I asked Dr. McConnell, "Can you call Greg and let him know how the surgery went?" Instantly, I realized that Greg, who I had also listed as my emergency contact, was a special part of my life.

Six months later, I walked down the aisle to marry my best friend. Two hearts healed by the power of love.

♥ *Vanessa Bruce Ingold*

# Planning for Major Health Events

A heart attack, days in the hospital and weeks recuperating at home will undoubtedly create chaos in your life. Plan now for any major life-changing, life-threatening event. Take control for yourself and your family.

- **Create a "find" list.** Include where to find your will, advance directive (living will) and organ donor card. List your bank accounts, safe deposit boxes, investments and key people such as your doctors, lawyer, accountant, insurance agent, stockbroker, relatives and anyone else who figures prominently in your family and business life. Give this list in a sealed envelope to the person who holds your designated power of attorney. Instruct that person to open the envelope only in the event of a medical emergency.
- **File important papers.** Where do you keep your insurance policies? Passport? Birth certificate? Other important papers? If you don't use a safe deposit box, buy a home safe (tell someone the combination) or store items in your freezer (safe from fire damage).
- **Appoint a power of attorney.** Appoint someone you can trust to act on your behalf if you

become incapacitated, if you're facing tricky surgery or if you become ill and cannot make decisions for yourself.

- **Update your will.** Make sure your affairs are in order and your most current will is on file with your attorney and anyone in your family who needs to know.
- **Sign an advance directive and appoint a health-care power of attorney.** An advance directive (living will) tells your relatives your wishes if you should be unable to make medical decisions for yourself. Do you want lifesaving measures to be taken? Do you want to be on life support? Do you wish nature to take its course? Do you want to donate your organs? Who will decide? Name the people you want to make that decision, and discuss your wishes with them in person, too.
- **Decide if you wish to be an organ donor, sign a donor card, put it in your purse or wallet and tell your family your wishes.**
- **Remember your loved ones.** This is the moment when you look into your heart, when you'll realize what is important and who really matters to you.

## Checklist: Vital Information

Items to file in a binder:

- ♥ Surgical and pathology reports and other vital medical records (such as lab results)
- ♥ All doctors' names and contact information
- ♥ Names of all medications (how much, how often) and the name of your pharmacy
- ♥ Blood pressure readings over time
- ♥ Copy of current EKG (carry a miniature version of this in your wallet or purse, too)
- ♥ Weight
- ♥ Insurance carrier

If you live alone, put a copy of your doctors' names and a list of all medications in an envelope and tape it near your phone in case of emergency. Ambulance personnel may find it useful if you cannot speak for yourself.

♥

## Dying Was Never an Option

*Sometimes we are to guard our heart . . .*
*protect it from invasion and*
*keep things safe and secure.*
*Sometimes we should give our heart . . .*
*let certain qualities out and release them to others.*

—CHARLES SWINDOLL

"Hi, I'm Sherry. I've had a heart transplant," I tell people at the health fair booth, where I volunteer for the Tennessee Donor Services.

"You're the first person I've ever met with a heart transplant," they always tell me. "You don't look different." And then they bring other people to come look at me.

I didn't feel different at age forty-nine in 1996 on a snowy Sunday morning in January. Until I felt a sudden crushing pain in my chest. I took two aspirin and lay down, waiting for the pain to go away. Surely I wasn't having a heart attack. Just two weeks earlier my doctor assessed my heart risk factors, and my cholesterol and blood pressure were just fine.

"You're having a heart attack," the ER doctor told me after my husband, Don, rushed me in the snowstorm to the local hospital. I began to protest, because dying was not an option, but I didn't remember anything else until a week later.

"Mother, you've had a heart transplant," my daughter Shannon was telling me through the fog of an anesthesia-induced coma.

Two IV poles were loaded with bags connected to tubes that were connected to me. Wires ran straight out of my body to an external pacemaker. I had the mandatory heart monitor and a chest tube coming out of my right lung. A heart transplant. No wonder I felt like I had been run over by an eighteen-wheeler.

Events of the previous week came to me in bits and pieces as family members told me what happened. The continuing snowstorm had grounded the medevac helicopter for two critical days, so I was taken by ambulance eighty miles to Vanderbilt University Hospital on the one open lane on the freeway.

I was immediately rushed to surgery to be put on a left ventricular assist device (LVAD). My husband, who had had no sleep since Sunday morning, and my two daughters, Tammy and Shannon, were told the only thing that would save me would be a heart transplant. My family was interviewed to qualify me for a transplant.

My condition was very critical. Chances of

finding a heart in a short time were slim, but doctors put me at the top of the transplant list anyway. They felt I would probably only last another twenty-four hours on these machines.

Yet in just hours—the shortest time ever to be on a transplant list—someone else's tragedy saved my life.

My family was told, "Prepare for the worst; it will take a miracle." Miracle indeed. Despite the snowstorm, my surgeon, Dr. Richard N. Pierson III, chartered a small jet and flew to Johnson City, Tennessee, to recover the heart himself. My donor was a twenty-two-year-old girl who had died from a brain aneurysm; that's all I have ever been told.

After retrieving the heart, the ambulance taking Dr. Pierson and the heart from the hospital back to the plane got stuck in the snow. There is a small window of time that a heart can still be viable— just four to six hours.

But luck was still on my side. The ambulance got through. Surgery expected to last up to ten hours took just four. The heart I received was larger than the heart I had. I learned that you could receive a larger heart but not a smaller heart, which worked in my favor because I am a small person. My transplant cardiologist, Dr. Stacy Davis, put it this way, "We took out a 350 engine and put in a 450 engine."

Transplant patients began coming to my room, sent by my doctor. They gave me information, but most of all, they gave me hope. I asked my doctor about my life expectancy and was told that they really don't know. They haven't been doing heart transplants long enough to determine that—especially in women. Most heart transplant patients are men.

After two months of complications with a miraculous recovery, I finally left Vanderbilt to an emotional homecoming. My house was filled with balloon bouquets, and our long driveway was festooned with yellow ribbons.

Having someone else's heart in my body was a strange feeling at first. It didn't feel like mine. I could feel every beat. I could see the beat by watching my clothing move. Sometimes at night while trying to go to sleep, it felt like it was going to beat right out of my chest. Eventually it became my heart. It skips a beat every now and then, but I'm used to it.

During a transplant, the nerves to my heart were cut; therefore, my new heart doesn't get the message from my brain to beat faster when I exercise or even get up to walk after sitting. Eventually it starts to beat faster. The reverse happens when I quit exercising. My heart continues to beat faster for a few minutes until it catches on that I have slowed down.

So I wondered if I could actually feel love coming from my heart. When my first grandchild was born, there it was—that familiar feeling of love coming right from my heart. Yes, this is definitely my heart now.

I wrote a thank-you letter to my donor family through the donor services, hoping they would write back and maybe even want to meet me. So far they haven't responded, but I'm still hoping. I know this was a very painful experience for them, but I want them to know they brought much joy to my family in their grief, as I'm sure they did to the other organ recipients. I want them to know I have taken very good care of this heart, and if it wasn't for them I wouldn't be alive.

Every single day is a gift. And every January 10 I celebrate a "re-birthday" with a red rose from my husband—one for every year since the transplant. I'm still basically the same person I was, but I appreciate small things more, am upbeat every day regardless of what happens. After all, today is a bonus day.

♥ *Sherry Shockley*

# Resources

## Organizations

**Heart and Stroke Foundation of Canada**, *www. heartandstroke.ca*, a national voluntary non-profit organization dedicated to preventing and reducing disability and death from heart disease and stroke through research, health promotion and advocacy.

**National Stroke Association**, *www.stroke.org*, (800) STROKES, a national non-profit organization that provides prevention, education and community programs.

**Women's Health Bureau**, *www.hc-sc.gc.ca/english/women/ resources.htm*, provides a series of fact sheets on heart health and gender.

**Harvard Center for Cancer Prevention:** Check your risk for heart disease at *www.yourdiseaserisk.harvard.edu*. You will be prompted to fill out brief questionnaires, and you will then get descriptions of your risk in the form of a coloured bar graph. The bar graph is a seven-level scale that compares you to typical men or women your age. You can click on personalized strategies to learn where to focus your prevention efforts and how to make lifestyle changes. With each click, the bar graph shrinks, and you can watch your risk drop.

**National Cholesterol Education Program:** Access the Risk Assessment Tool for Estimating Your Ten-Year Risk of Having a Heart Attack at *http://hin.nhlbi.nih.gov/atpiii/calculator.asp?usertype=pub*. The risk assessment tool uses information from the Framingham Heart Study to predict a person's chance of having a heart attack in the next ten years. This tool is designed for adults aged twenty and older who do not have heart disease or diabetes. To find your risk score, enter your information in the calculator.

**National Heart, Lung, and Blood Institute,** a division of the National Institutes of Health, in the Department of Health and Human Services, at *www.nhlbi.nih.gov*

- Heart and Vascular Diseases, information for patients and the public at *www.nhlbi.nih.gov/health/public/heart/index.htm#chol*

- Facts about the DASH Eating Plan at *www.nhlbi.nih.gov/health/public/heart/hbp/dash/index.htm*

- The Heart Truth, a national awareness campaign about women and heart disease sponsored by the National Heart, Lung, and Blood Institute at *www.nhlbi.nih.gov/health/hearttruth*

- Act in Time to Heart Attack Signs, a national awareness campaign, at *www.nhlbi.nih.gov/actintime/index.htm*

**National Center for Early Defibrillation**, (866) AED-INFO, *www.early-defib.org*

**United Network for Organ Sharing (UNOS)**, a non-profit organization under contract by the Department of Health and Human Services to operate the Organ Procurement and Transplantation Network and to develop a national system to assure equal access for all patients needing organs at *www.optn.org.*

**Coalition on Donation**, a nonprofit alliance of major professional, patient, health, science, transplant and voluntary organizations dedicated to increasing public awareness on organ and tissue donation at *www.shareyourlife.org* .

**Centre for Chronic Disease Prevention and Control Cardiovascular Disease**, provides publications, statistics, and definitions. Contact them at:

Public Health Agency of Canada
130 Colonnade Road
A.L. 6501H
Ottawa, ON K1A 0K9
*www.phac-aspc.gc.ca*

## Supporting Organization

### The Hope Heart Institute:
### a pioneering leader in heart disease
### research, education and prevention

The Hope Heart Institute ("The Hope") is a nonprofit organization that has been on the forefront of cardiovascular research, education and prevention for more than forty-five years.

Named after Bob Hope, who lent his name and support in the early 1980s, The Hope is dedicated to preventing and treating heart and blood vessel disease and to improving the physical, emotional and spiritual quality of life for all who are at risk of, or afflicted with, cardiovascular disease.

World-renowned cardiovascular surgeon and research scientist Lester R. Sauvage, M.D., established The Hope Heart Institute in Seattle, Washington, to help those suffering from the devastating effects of cardiovascular disease. Soon, he and his team earned international recognition by pioneering coronary artery bypass graft surgery—still the most frequently performed heart operation in the world.

One of the many exciting projects under way in

The Hope Heart Program at the Benaroya Research Institute is the "living heart": a $10 million project funded by the National Institutes of Health to grow a patch of heart tissue that may lead, someday, to growing an entire heart from a patient's own cells. Researchers at The Hope are developing noninvasive methods of treating problems in the heart, blood vessels and other organs, perhaps replacing surgery.

The Hope Health division is the industry leader in health and wellness publications and publisher of the highly acclaimed *HOPE Health Letter*. Widely distributed to employees through their employers, it is read by more than five million people each month. Much of the heart health content in this book was supplied by Hope Health.

Education programs at The Hope include an organ donor program, educational workshops for women, and a curriculum for students from kindergarten through twelfth grade to teach them the value of a healthy heart and healthy lifestyle.

The Hope relies on publication revenues, government grants, research contracts and private donations to operate. For more information, contact The Hope at (206) 903-2001 or visit *www.HopeHeart.org*.

## Who Is Jack Canfield, Co-creator of *Chicken Soup for the Soul*®?

**Jack Canfield** is one of America's leading experts in the development of human potential and personal effectiveness. He is both a dynamic, entertaining speaker and a highly sought-after trainer. Jack has a wonderful ability to inform and inspire audiences toward increased levels of self-esteem and peak performance. He has authored or coauthored numerous books, including *Dare to Win, The Aladdin Factor, 100 Ways to Build Self-Concept in the Classroom, Heart at Work* and *The Power of Focus.* His latest book is *The Success Principles.*

*www.jackcanfield.com*

## Who is Mark Victor Hansen, Co-creator of *Chicken Soup for the Soul*®?

In the area of human potential, no one is more respected than **Mark Victor Hansen**. For more than thirty years, Mark has focused solely on helping people from all walks of life reshape their personal vision of what's possible. His powerful messages of possibility, opportunity and action have created powerful change in thousands of organizations and millions of individuals worldwide. He is a prolific writer of bestselling books such as *The One Minute Millionaire, The Power of Focus, The Aladdin Factor* and *Dare to Win.*

*www.markvictorhansen.com*

## Who Is Vicki Rackner, M.D.?

**Vicki Rackner, M.D., F.A.C.S.**, is a board-certified surgeon and clinical faculty member at the University of Washington School of Medicine. She is the medical editor of *The HOPE Health Letter* and serves on the Medical Advisory Board of The Hope Heart Institute. She is an author, speaker and member of the National Speakers Association. She left the operating room to be on the cutting edge of health-care consumerism, and she is now a full-time patient advocate through her company Medical Bridges (*www.MedicalBridges.com*), which focuses on offering bridges: the bridge between patient and doctor, the bridge between employer and employee, and the bridge between lifestyle and health. Most importantly, she offers the bridge between the health care patients get and the health care they want.

## Who Is Sandra J. Wendel (writer)?

**Sandra J. Wendel**, a consumer-health writer and editor, collaborated with Dr. Edward Creagan, a cancer specialist at Mayo Clinic, on the book *How Not to Be My Patient*. She develops health content for *eMedicineHealth.com* and her own company's online health content at *www.Health-eHeadlines.com*. She is editor of the *Wise Women Speak* book series, *www.wise-woman-health.com*.

# Sources

**The Hope Heart Institute** (*www.HopeHeart.org*), medical expertise for health information. Thanks to Thomas Amidon, M.D., F.A.C.C., Medical Director of The Hope Heart Institute; Mark Nudelman, Executive Vice President; Jamie R. Jensen, Director of Marketing. Pioneering cardiovascular surgeon Lester R. Sauvage, M.D., founded The Hope Heart Institute in 1959.

**Hope Health** (*www.HopeHealth.com*), a health-based communication company specializing in producing information distributed at workplaces. Publishes a variety of lifestyle-related information, including the award-winning *The HOPE Health Letter*, the most widely circulated employee health letter. Proceeds from sales of health information go to support the research efforts of The Hope Heart Institute.

*Is It Worth Dying For? A Self-Assessment Program to Make Stress Work for You, Not Against You* by Robert Eliot, M.D., with Dennis Breo (Bantam, 1991).

*From Stress to Strength: How to Lighten Your Load and Save Your Life* by Robert Eliot, M.D. (Bantam, 1995).

*The Open Heart: Secret to Happiness*, Lester R. Sauvage, M.D. (Better Life Press, 1998).

*You Can Beat Heart Disease: Prevention and Treatment*, Lester R. Sauvage, M.D. (Better Life Press, 1998).

*The Better Life Diet: A Simple Plan for a Long and Youthful Life*, Lester R. Sauvage, M.D., with Robert H. Knopp, M.D. (Better Life Press, 2000).

*Thriving with Heart Disease: Live Happier, Healthier, Longer*, Wayne M. Sotile, Ph.D. with Robin Cantor-Cooke (Free Press, 2003).

# Contributors

**Banjo Bandolas**'s stories have been published in numerous regional and national publications. His style of storytelling reflects and remains true to his southern roots. Previous anthologies include *Dead on Demand, Chicken Soup for the Fisherman's Soul, Ghosts at the Coasts* and the upcoming *Chicken Soup for the Fisherman's Soul II.* Currently, he lives the good life in Eugene, Oregon. You can e-mail him at *banjo@real-beer.com.*

**Deborah D. Coble** is a New York publicist originally from Memphis, Tennessee. Her work with Project Kids Worldwide, *www.projectkidsworldwide.org,* resulted in international media coverage of a 9/11 widow raising money to sponsor children for lifesaving heart surgery in her husband's memory. Deborah plans on writing a book about her experience in New York and can be reached at *ddcoble@aol.com.*

**Tracey Conway** is an Emmy–award-winning actress and nominated writer and an internationally known professional speaker. With a career spanning live theater, television and independent feature film, Tracey continues to enjoy a wide variety of performing challenges, but is proudest to have made an appearance on *Oprah* to tell her story of sudden cardiac arrest. When not traveling the world presenting her survival story, *Drop Dead Gorgeous!* she makes her home in Seattle with her furry Siberian husky "daughter," Lulu Eloise la Diablita (the little devil girl). She is a member of the board of The Hope Heart Institute. Tracey can be reached through her Web site *www.traceyconway.com.*

After twenty-five years as an Air Force wife, **Twink DeWitt**—with her husband, Denny—serve ten years with Mercy Ships. They work with training schools and writers' schools for Youth With a Mission in Hawaii and Texas. Together, the DeWitts founded Heritage Anchor to help others write family stories that become legacies for future generations. She has been published in previous *Chicken Soup for the Soul* books and has written for *LifeWise Magazine* and Walk Thru the Bible's *Tapestry*. The DeWitts have three married sons and five grandchildren. They can be reached at *dewitt@tyler.net*.

**Mark Christopher Drury** is a man on a mission to lose 250 pounds. His speeches explode with his tales of self-discovery and reMARKable successes as he approaches that staggering goal. He has been featured in *The Leanness Lifestyle,* has co-authored three books of inspiration and humor, and is the author of his own story triumph, *The Weigh Out.* Mark tells of going from 422 pounds to appearing on radio and television, aerobic certification, parasailing, singing, speaking, bodybuilding competition and an ever-widening array of once-impossible goals. E-mail Mark at *markdrury@markgetsitdone.com* or through his Web site at *www.markgetsitdone.com*.

Hailed as the Erma Bombeck for the twenty-first century, **Rudy Wilson Galdonik** is the author of *Take Heart! True Stories of Life, Love, and Laughter.* She is a lifelong heart patient with $40,000 worth of "stuff" in her chest. She works with organizations that want to empower individuals to use humor as a way to manage stress, enhance creativity and increase effectiveness. Rudy is also the cochair of the American Heart Association's Women and Heart Disease Committee, Southeastern New England and a member of the board of directors of the Adult Congenital Heart Association. She can be reached via her Web site: *www.Rudywg.com*.

In 1992 **Bonnie Compton Hanson** and her husband, Don, were busy with church and community service, their careers, children, grandchildren, pets and garden. Bonnie authored several books. Don was a senior systems analyst, working around the clock. Then it happened. Because of all they went through—finally finding hope through a "generator" and daily medication—they want to share their heart story with others. Contact Bonnie and Don at *bonnieh1@worldnet.att.net*.

**Vanessa Bruce Ingold** was run over by a truck at age twenty-three, while bicycle riding. Now being called a "Walking Miracle," she has articles in books such as *Nudges from God* (Obadiah Press) and *Sharing Visions* (CSS Publishing). Vanessa and husband Greg live in Southern California. Contact her at *JCnessa@aol.com*.

**Jann Mitchell** is an American writer living in Stockholm, Sweden. Her books include *Home Sweeter Home* and *Love Sweeter Love;* her work is featured in the *Chicken Soup for the Soul* series and other anthologies. She travels widely and sponsors a day-care center in Tanzania, East Africa, but still makes it back to the United States several times yearly to visit her children, grandchildren and very special sisters. Reach her at *jannmmitchell@aol.com*.

**Jan Richardson** has been redesigning her life since her triple bypass surgery in May 2002. She has been rediscovering her love for the creative side of life—writing and interior decorating—and is an active community volunteer. Jan shares her story with others through speaking, in hopes of helping other women make necessary changes in their lives. Jan owned her own business before getting "kicked off the merry-go-round," providing administrative and marketing support for a variety of entrepreneurs, including Kay Allenbaugh, creator/author of the national bestselling series *Chocolate for a Woman's Soul*. In December 2003, Jan took a position as the director for Civic Outreach, Inc., welcoming executive leadership to her community in Tigard, Oregon. Contact Jan at *jan@speakersolutions.net*.

**Sallie Rodman** is a freelance writer residing in Los Alamitos, California, with her husband, a dog and a cat. She has a certificate in professional writing from California State University, Long Beach. Her work has appeared in *Chicken Soup for the Mother & Daughter Soul*, *Chocolate for a Woman's Courage* and various magazines and newspapers. She is currently working on her own story, *Panic Demons: My Life with Panic Attacks and Agoraphobia*. You may reach her at *srodman@ix.netcom.com*.

**Sherry Shockley** lives in Cookeville, Tennessee, with her husband of forty years, Don. She is a happy grandmother and mother of two daughters—Tammy, a nurse practitioner in women's health, and Shannon, a pharmacist who specializes in transplant medicine. She's fond of saying, "What a mother won't do for her child's career!" She was working at Tennessee Technological University as a secretary at the time of her heart transplant. She enjoys gardening, camping and reading, but most importantly, volunteers for Tennessee Donor Services and Mended Hearts—a local affiliate of the American Heart Association that offers the gift of hope to heart patients and their families (*www.mendedhearts.org*).

**Ruth Vance** is the mother of three, the grandmother of two and, thankfully, the wife of one still active husband. She lives in Huntsville, Alabama.

**Kimberly Zweygardt**, a certified registered nurse anesthetist, is the owner of Moonlight Anesthesia, PA, providing anesthesia for rural hospitals in Kansas, Colorado and Nebraska. She is a 1979 graduate of St. Francis Hospital School of Nursing, Wichita, Kansas, and graduated in 1983 from Samford University/ Baptist Medical Centers School of Anesthesia, Birmingham, Alabama. Kim is also a writer, speaker and dramatist portraying women from the Bible with Lamplight Ministries. Family time is spent with husband, Kary, sons, Jordan and Britt, daughter, Lauren, and dogs, Inky, Molly, Dozer and Lucy, plus Clifford, the big red cat. Hobbies include napping, writing, travel and cooking. Contact her at *www.kimzweygardt.com*.

## Permissions *(continued from page ii)*

*Kicked Off the Merry-Go-Round* reprinted by permission Jan Richardson from "Wise Women Speak: Stepping Stones Along the Path" ©2003 Jan Richardson.

*Singing His Heart Out* reprinted by permission Bonnie Compton Hanson. ©2004 Bonnie Compton Hanson.

*Serious as a Heart Attack* reprinted by permission Banjo Bandolas. ©1999 Banjo Bandolas.

*Mission Possible: Healing One Heart from Baghdad* reprinted by permission Deborah D. Coble. ©2004 Deborah D. Coble.

*How to Meditate* reprinted by permission The Women's Heart Foundation. ©1993 The Women's Heart Foundation, *www.womensheart.org.*

*In a Heartbeat* reprinted by permission Kimberly Zweygardt, CRNA. ©2004 Kimberly Zweygardt, CRNA.

*A Shocking Start* reprinted by permission Ford Hudson and Thomas Crandall. ©2004 Ford Hudson and Thomas Crandall.

*Thanks for the Miracle, Sis* reprinted by permission Jann M. Mitchell. ©1993 Jann M. Mitchell. Previously published in *The Oregonian* and *Chocolate for a Woman's Soul* ©1997 Fireside, a division of Simon & Schuster.

*Cradled in God's Hands* reprinted by permission Sallie Rodman. ©2004 Sallie Rodman.

*A Damaged Heart Finds Love* reprinted by permission Vanessa Bruce Ingold. ©2004 Vanessa Bruce Ingold.

*Dying Was Never an Option* reprinted by permission Sherry Shockley. ©2004 Sherry Shockley.

*The Struggle Index* reprinted from "From Stress to Strength: How to Lighten Your Load and Save Your Life," Robert S. Eliot, M.D., Bantam, Doubleday Dell. ©1994 Robert S. Eliot, M.D. Rights owned and controlled by Mrs. Phyllis Eliot. Reprinted with permission.

# NOTES

# Just what the doctor ordered...

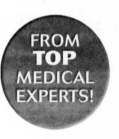

## Look for these
## great topics in the

*Chicken Soup for the Soul®*
*Healthy Living Series*

Arthritis
Asthma
Breast Cancer
Depression
Diabetes
Heart Disease
Menopause
Back Pain
Stress
Weight Loss

FROM
**TOP**
MEDICAL
EXPERTS!

For more information or to submit stories
please visit
**www.thehealthysoul.com**

To order by telephone (800) 441-5569